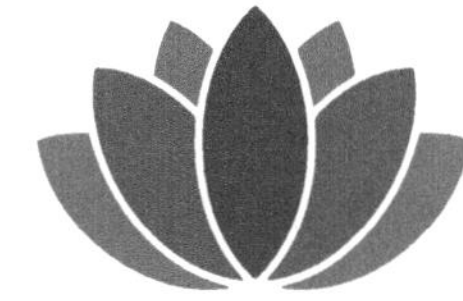

THE HOLISTIC GUITARIST

A COMPLETE GUIDE TO MUSICAL WELL-BEING

SEAN McGOWAN

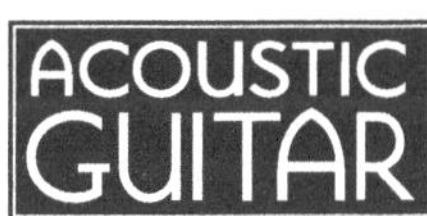

Publisher: Lyzy Lusterman
Editor: Adam Perlmutter
Managing Editor: Stephanie Campos Dal Broi
Copyeditor: E.E. Bradman
Music Proofreader: Mark Althans
Design and Production: Joey Lusterman

ISBN 978-1-936604-50-0

Printed in the United States of America

This book was produced by String Letter Publishing, Inc.
330 Sir Francis Drake Boulevard, Suite K, San Anselmo, CA 94960
(510) 215-0010; Stringletter.com

Library of Congress Control Number: 2025936208

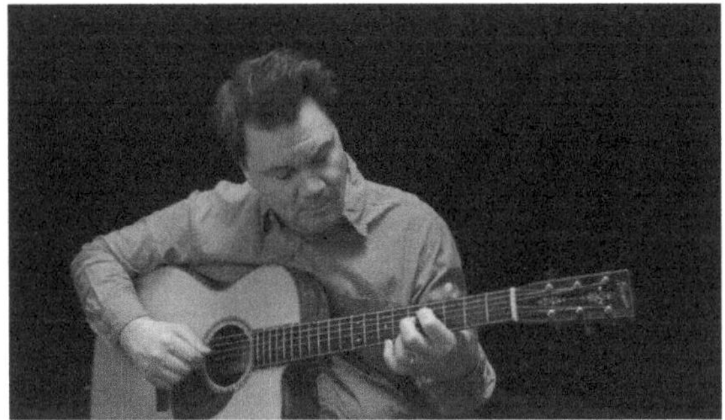

Video downloads to accompany the lessons and preludes in this book are available at **store.acousticguitar.com/holisticvideo**

Introduction

How do accomplished guitarists practice? What do they work on, and for how long? How do they practice difficult and advanced material and never get injured? Or do they? Is it possible to sustain a lifelong commitment to playing the guitar, while continually striving to get better, discover new music, widen your abilities, and do it without incident? These are questions I've been asking myself and working to answer for the better part of the last thirty years. The short answer to these questions, by the way, is yes. Absolutely!

The Backstory

Many years ago, I was a college student trying to find my place and musical identity in the world, especially within my school and local communities as a guitarist. As someone who had to work to fund my education, school was a long journey. It took me roughly ten years and stints at three different institutions to earn my undergraduate degree in music. My experience as a college student included working non-musical jobs, constantly performing, traveling for gigs, teaching, and practicing. In hindsight, being forced to balance classroom learning and bandstand education was a gift.

I eventually earned my bachelor's degree from Berklee College of Music in Boston. By the time I started there, I was 26 and already had years of professional experience as a player and teacher. Besides the incredible abundance of talent, hard work, and dedication at Berklee, there were also injuries, anxiety, and a general sense of unhappiness that no one ever addressed in the classroom or studio.

Up until that point, I had never encountered a guitar teacher that talked about how to play the guitar from the standpoint of good posture, relaxation techniques, and preventing overuse injuries. Conversely, there was a sense, perhaps subconscious, that the harder students practiced, the more they improved and received palpable benefits (e.g., gigs, recognition, respect, grades, etc.). Subsequently, I noticed many students—as well as faculty—suffering from overuse injuries such as tendonitis and carpal tunnel. But no one ever seemed to talk about it.

Fortunately, while at Berklee, I met people and discovered resources that totally changed my trajectory and approach to playing the guitar and music. Richard Ehrman was a musician and certified Feldenkrais practitioner who was on staff at Berklee in the 1990s, and he offered free Feldenkrais/Awareness Through Movement classes, open to all students and faculty.

Every class was a breakthrough in understanding how to interface my body with movement and playing my instrument. At the same time, I attended Alexander Technique workshops at Boston Conservatory and witnessed how this methodology really improved the posture, tone, and clarity of classical string players.

I also took classes with guitar teacher/tai chi practitioner Joe Rogers, who taught a George Van Eps guitar lab and seamlessly integrated principles of meditation, breathwork, patience, and qigong into every class. Rogers was able to bring calmness and peace to the classroom, offering a respite from a fast-paced urban environment that always demanded one's energy. He did this by allowing us the chance to take everything slowly and with solid concentration. This may seem obvious, but it's rare that we give ourselves the gift of slowing down.

These experiences had a profound impact on my sense of well-being and my approach to playing. Three books published in the 1990s—*You Are Your Instrument* by Julie Lyonn Lieberman, *The Art of Practicing* by Madeline Bruser, and *Effortless Mastery* by Kenny Werner— also helped shape my teaching and practicing trajectories. As a college student living in a large urban city, *Effortless*

Mastery was an indispensable resource that I consulted often. Throughout the book, Werner, a noted jazz pianist, describes being a student, practicing, and thriving as a professional musician with refreshing nuance and excruciating detail, and I completely related to his story. Fortunately, there is now an *Effortless Mastery Institute* at Berklee, and strategies of injury prevention, body awareness, and creative fulfillment, are now thankfully addressed and explored at higher education programs across the United States and Canada.

In addition to playing with lots of different bands and exploring diverse styles of music in the 1990s, I played solo guitar accompanying modern dance companies. It was incredible to work with non-musicians who—despite having a visceral approach to and keen awareness of music—didn't communicate using musical terms. Some of what we did was completely improvised, while other performances were through-composed to choreography.

What I noticed was a big difference between the lifestyles of dancers and how they prepared for performances with those of typical musicians. Dancers were acutely aware of maintaining their bodies—in effect, their instruments—through conditioning, nutrition, and various bodywork modalities such as yoga, Pilates, and massage. They would typically arrive hours before a performance, sometimes running the entire show as a rehearsal/warm-up, and took great care to physically stretch and mentally prepare for the performance.

Embracing Music as a Holistic Endeavor

Several years ago, I developed The Holistic Musician, a course at the University of Colorado Denver, where I have served as a music professor since 2007. Open to all instrumentalists and vocalists, this class surveys the most common idiosyncratic injuries, by instrument, among practicing and professional musicians, as well as prevention strategies and maintenance techniques.

The course also explores two topics not often addressed in music education: mental wellness

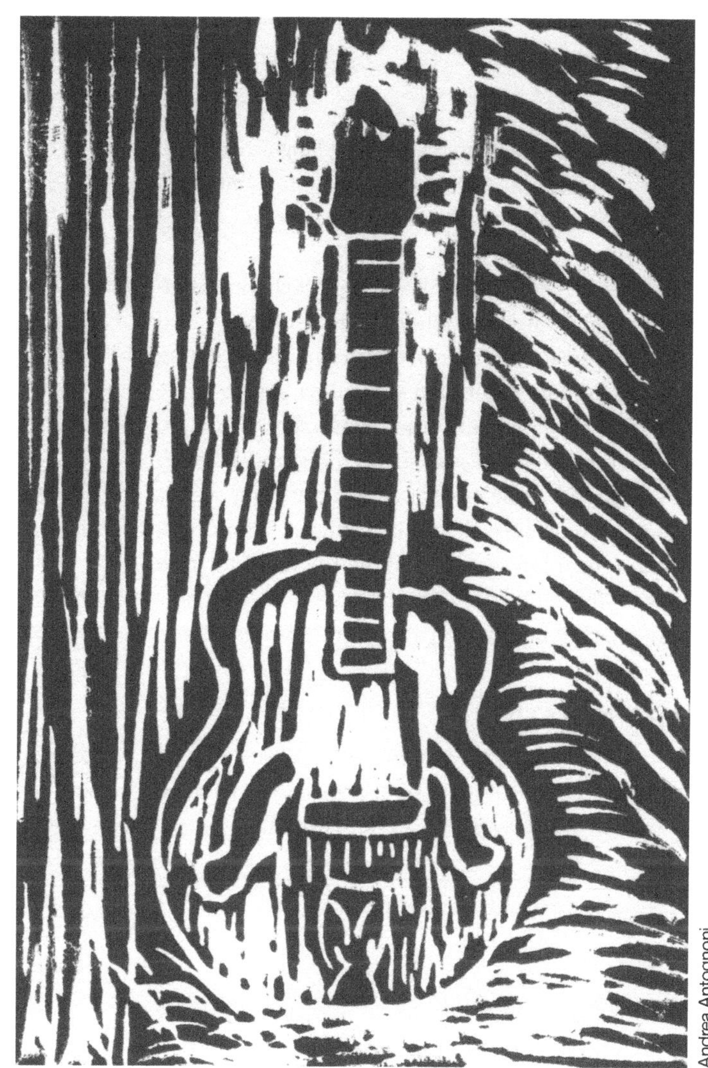

Andrea Antognoni

and musical well-being. As a class, we study various methodologies that have proven successful for musicians, including Alexander Technique, Feldenkrais, yoga, biofeedback, organized practice journals, and hearing protection, and we focus on methods of preventing injuries and promoting mental stability, which can be cultivated and practiced just like a piece of music.

In conceiving of this book specifically for guitarists, my ongoing mantra was, "Write a book you want to read; write a book that people need." I sincerely hope that this book inspires, offers a creative spark, serves as a resource for injury prevention and care, and reminds readers how fortunate we are as guitarists and musicians. We've all shared the joy of learning an instrument, for the benefit of ourselves and others. It's been said that playing the guitar is the most affordable form of therapy. I know it has impacted my life and the lives of many others in such a positive and beautiful way. What else could we ask for?

—Sean McGowan

Notation Guide

Music is a language and, like many languages, has a written form. In order to be literate, one must become familiar with what each character and symbol represent.

Guitarists use several types of notation, including standard notation, tablature, and chord diagrams. Standard notation is a universal system in Western music. Becoming competent with standard notation will allow you to share and play music with almost any other instrument. Tablature is a notation system exclusively for stringed instruments with frets—like guitar and ukulele—that shows you what strings and frets to play to achieve the desired pitches. Chord diagrams use a graphic representation of the fretboard to show chord shapes on fretted instruments. Here's a primer on how to read these types of notation.

STANDARD NOTATION

Standard notation is written on a five-line staff. Notes are written in alphabetical order from A to G. Every time you pass a G note, the sequence of notes repeats, starting with A.

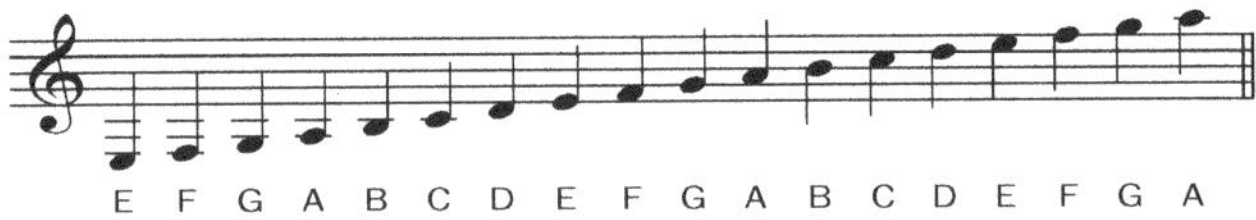

The duration of a note is depicted by note head, stem, and flag. Though the number of beats each note represents will vary depending on the meter, the relations between note durations remain the same: a whole note (𝅝) is double the length of a half note (𝅗𝅥). A half note is double the length of a quarter note (♩). A quarter note is double the length of an eighth note (♪). An eighth note is double the length of a sixteenth note (𝅘𝅥𝅯). And so on. You'll notice each time a flag gets added, the note duration halves.

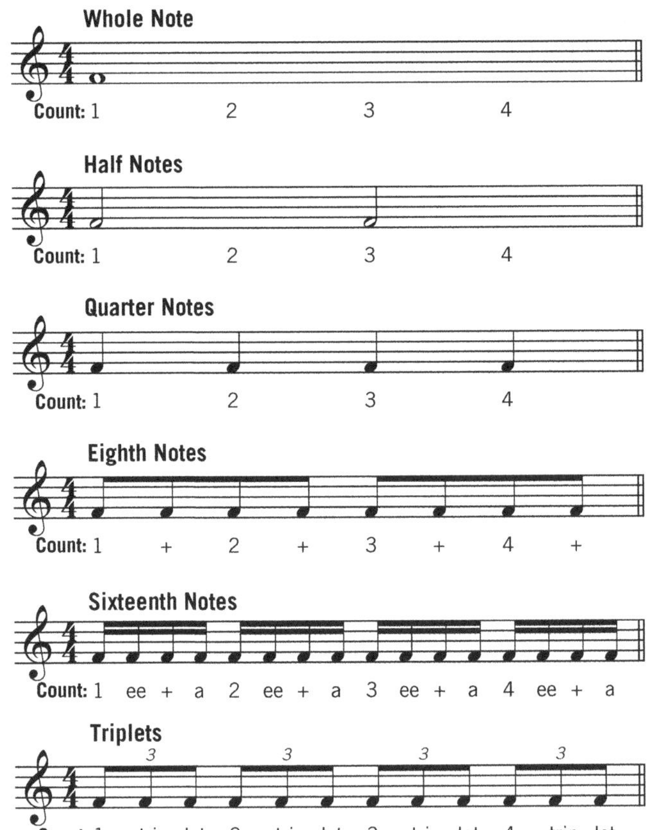

The numbers that follow the clef (4/4, 3/4, 6/8, etc.) or **C** shown at the beginning of a piece of music denote the time signature. The top number tells you how many beats are in each measure, and the bottom number indicates the rhythmic value of each beat (4 equals a quarter note, 8 equals an eighth note, 16 equals a sixteenth note, and 2 equals a half note).

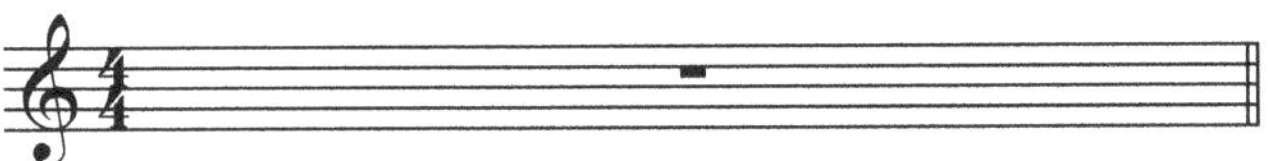

The most common time signature is 4/4, which signifies four quarter notes per measure and is sometimes designated with the symbol **C** (for common time). The symbol **¢** stands for cut time (2/2).

TABLATURE

In tablature, the six horizontal lines represent the six strings of the guitar, low to high, as on the guitar. The numbers refer to fret numbers on the indicated string.

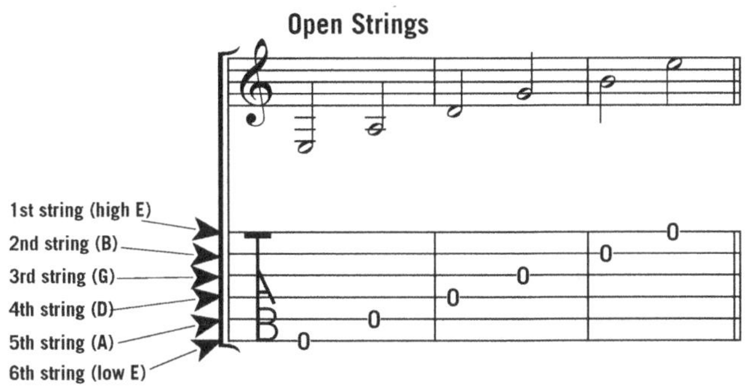

FINGERINGS

Fingerings are indicated with small numbers and letters in the notation. Fretting-hand fingering is expressed as 1 for the index finger, 2 the middle, 3 the ring, 4 the pinky, and *T* the thumb. Picking-hand fingering is conveyed by *i* for the index finger, *m* the middle, *a* the ring, *c* the pinky, and *p* the thumb.

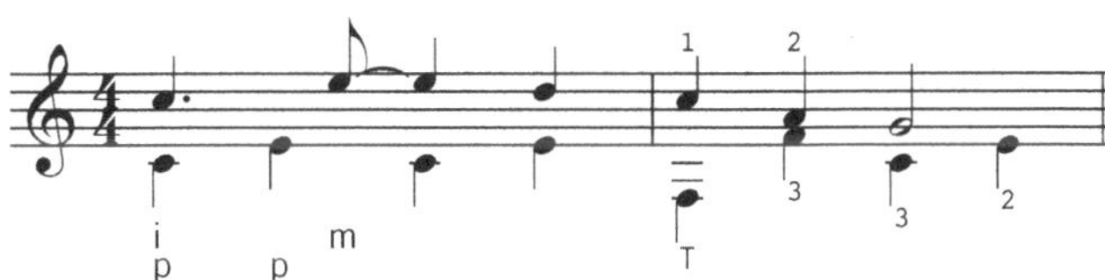

STRUMMING AND PICKING

In music played with a flatpick, downstrokes (toward the floor) and upstrokes (toward the ceiling) are shown as follows. Slashes in the notation and tablature indicate a strum through the previously played chord.

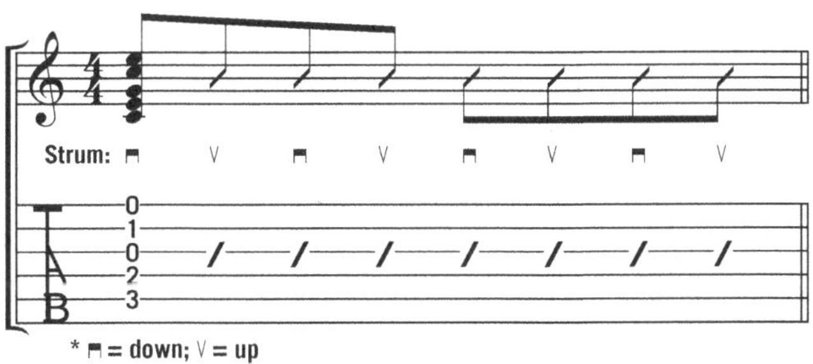

In music played with the pick-hand fingers, *split stems* are often used to highlight the division between thumb and fingers. With split stems, notes played by the thumb have stems pointing down, while notes played by the fingers have stems pointing up. If split stems are not used, pick-hand fingerings are usually present. Here is the same fingerpicking pattern shown with and without split stems. Clarity will inform which option is used.

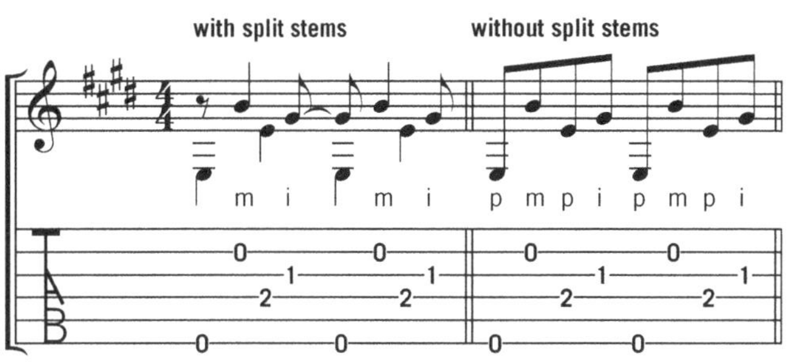

CHORD DIAGRAMS

Chord diagrams are a convenient way of depicting chord shapes. Frets are presented horizontally. The thick top line represents the nut. A fret number to the right of a diagram indicates a chord played higher up the neck (in this case the top horizontal line is thin and the fret number is designated). Strings are shown as vertical lines. The line on the far left represents the sixth (lowest) string, and the line on the far right represents the first (highest) string. Dots mark where the fingers go, and thick horizontal lines illustrate barres. Numbers above the diagram are fretting-hand finger numbers, as used in standard notation.

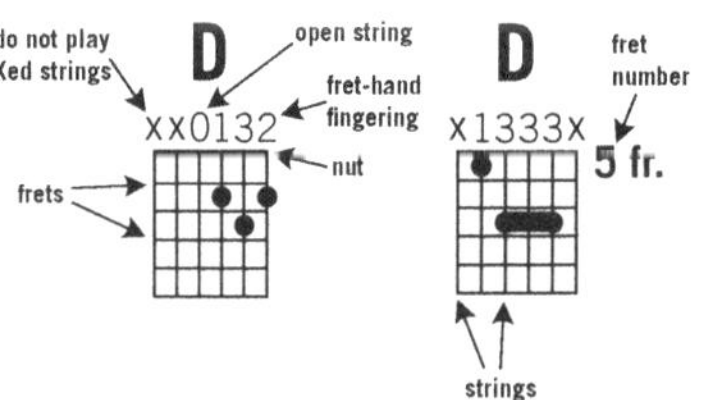

The given fingerings are only suggestions. They are generally what would most typically be considered standard. In context, however, musical passages may benefit from other fingerings for smoothest chord transitions. An X means a string that should be muted or not played; 0 indicates an open string.

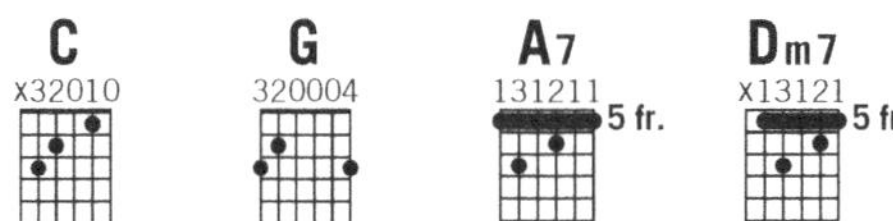

Notation Guide

CAPOS

If a capo is used, a Roman numeral designates the fret where the capo should be placed. The standard notation and tablature is written as if the capo were the nut of the guitar. For instance, a tune capoed anywhere up the neck and played using key-of-G chord shapes and fingerings will be written in the key of G. Likewise, open strings held down by the capo are written as open strings.

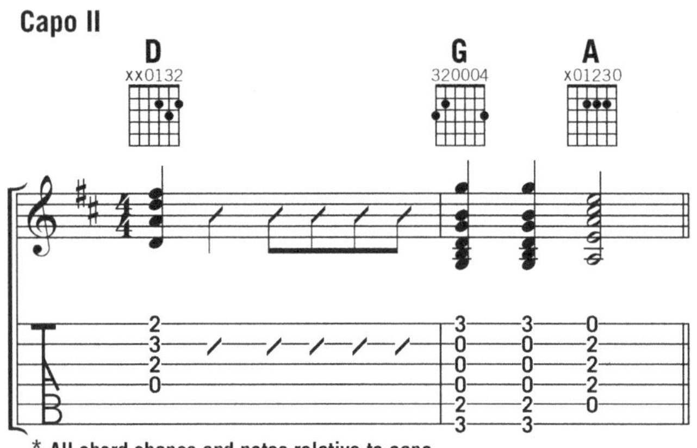

TUNINGS

Alternate tunings are given from the lowest (sixth) string to the highest (first) string. D A D G B E is standard tuning with the bottom string dropped to D. Standard notation for songs in alternate tunings always reflects the actual pitches of the notes.

VOCAL TUNES

Vocal tunes are sometimes written with a fully tabbed-out introduction and a vocal melody with chord diagrams for the rest of the piece. The tab intro is usually your clue as to which strumming or fingerpicking pattern to use in the rest of the piece. The melody with lyrics underneath is that which is sung by the vocalist. Occasionally, smaller notes are written with the melody to indicate other instruments or the harmony part sung by another vocalist. These are not to be confused with cue notes, which are small notes that express variation in melodies when a section is repeated. Listen to a recording of the piece to get a feel for the guitar accompaniment and to hear the singing if you aren't skilled at reading vocal melodies.

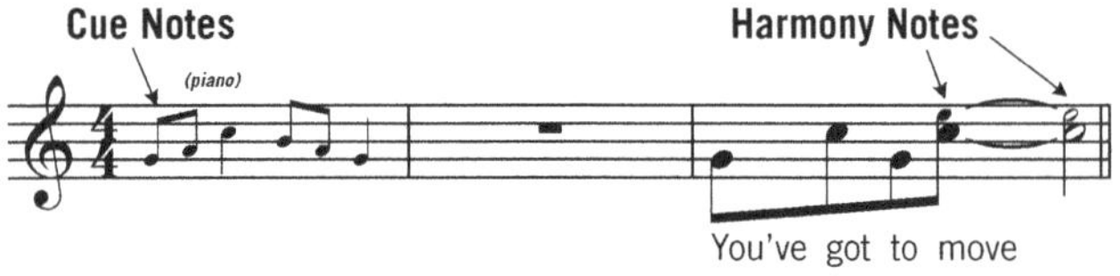

ARTICULATIONS

There are a number of ways you can articulate a note on the guitar. Notes connected with slurs (not to be confused with ties) in the tablature or standard notation are executed with either a hammer-on, pull-off, or slide. Lower notes slurred to higher notes are played as hammer-ons; higher notes slurred to lower notes are played as pull-offs.

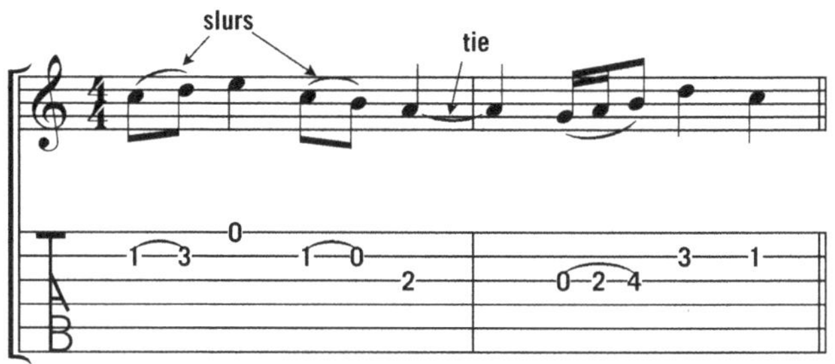

Slides are represented with dashes. A dash preceding a note is a slide into the note from an indefinite point in the direction of the slide; a dash following a note is a slide off the note to an indefinite point in the direction of the slide. For two slurred notes connected with a slide, pick the first note and then slide into the second.

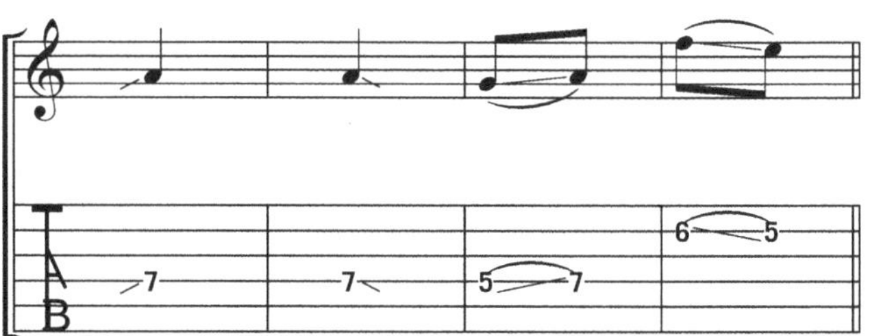

Bends are denoted with upward arrows. Most bends have a specific destination pitch—the number above the bend symbol shows how much the bend raises the pitch: ¼ for a slight bend, ½ for a half step, 1 for a whole step.

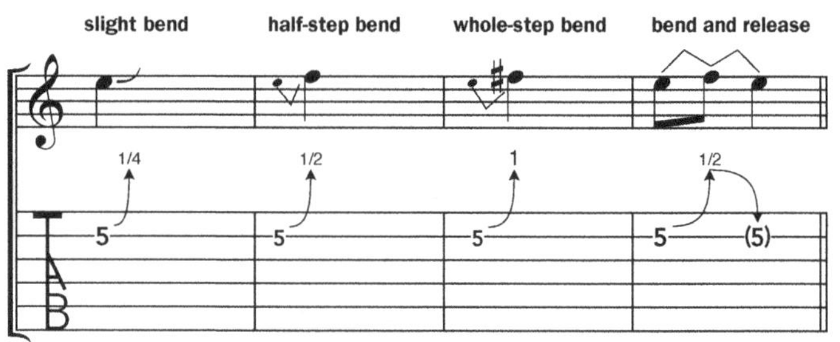

Grace notes are represented by small notes with a slash through the stem in standard notation and with small numbers in the tablature. A grace note is a quick musical ornament with no specific note value leading into a note, most commonly executed as a hammer-on, pull-off, or slide. In the first example below, pluck the note at the fifth fret on the beat, then quickly hammer onto the seventh fret. The second example is executed as a quick pull-off from the second fret to the open string. In the third example, both notes at the fifth fret are played simultaneously (even though it appears that the fourth string at the fifth fret is to be played by itself), then the fourth string, seventh fret is quickly hammered.

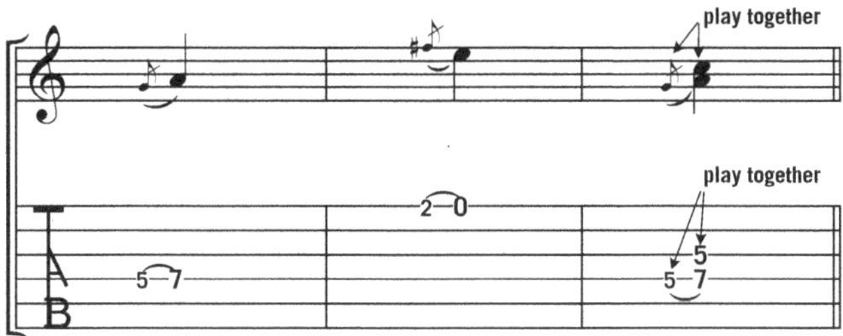

HARMONICS

Harmonics are expressed as diamond-shaped notes in the standard notation and a small dot next to the tablature numbers. Natural harmonics are indicated with the text "Harmonics" or "Harm." above the tablature. Harmonics articulated with the picking hand (often called artificial harmonics) include the text "R.H. Harmonics" or "R.H. Harm." above the tab. Picking-hand harmonics are executed by lightly touching the harmonic node (usually 12 frets above the open string or fretted note) with the picking hand index finger and plucking the string with the thumb, ring finger, or pick. For extended phrases played with picking-hand harmonics, the fretted notes are shown in the tab along with instructions to touch the harmonics 12 frets above the notes.

Touch harmonic
12 frets above note
Harm.
Harm.
Harm.
R. H. Harm.

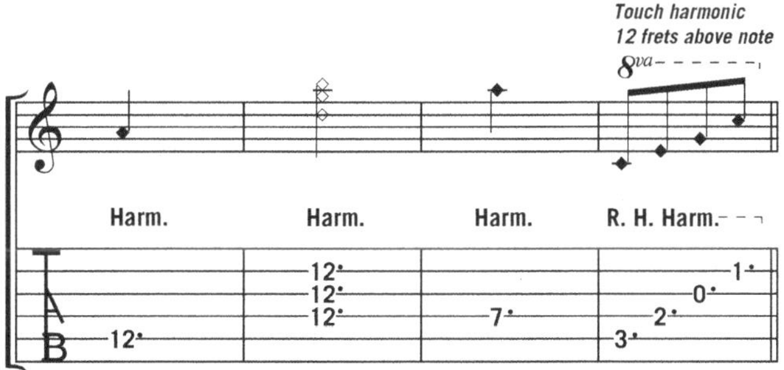

REPEATS

One of the most confusing parts of a musical score can be the navigation symbols, such as repeats, *D.S. al Coda*, *D.C. al Fine*, *To Coda*, etc. Repeat symbols are placed at the beginning and end of the passage to be repeated.

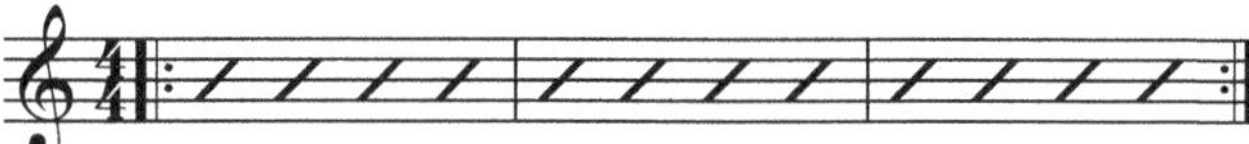

When you encounter a repeat sign, take note of the location of the begin repeat symbol (with the dots to the right of the lines), play until you reach the end repeat symbol (with the dots to the left of the lines). Then go back to the begin repeat sign, and play the section again.

If you find an end repeat only sign, go back to the beginning of the piece and repeat. The next time you get to the end repeat, continue to the next section of the piece unless there is text that specifically indicates to repeat additional times.

A section will often have a different ending after each repeat. The example below includes a first and a second ending. Play until you hit the repeat symbol, return to the begin repeat symbol, and play until you reach the bracketed first ending. Then skip the measures under the bracket and jump immediately to the second ending, and then continue.

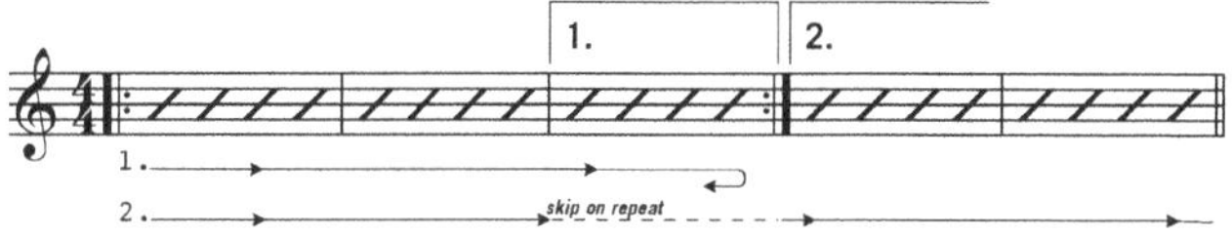

D.S. stands for *dal segno* or "from the sign." When you encounter this indication, advance immediately to the sign (𝄋). *D.S.* is usually accompanied by *al Fine* or *al Coda*. *Fine* indicates the end of a piece. A coda is a final passage near the end of a piece and is indicated with 𝄌. *D.S. al Coda* simply tells you to go back to the sign and continue on until you are instructed to move to the coda, indicated with *To Coda* 𝄌.

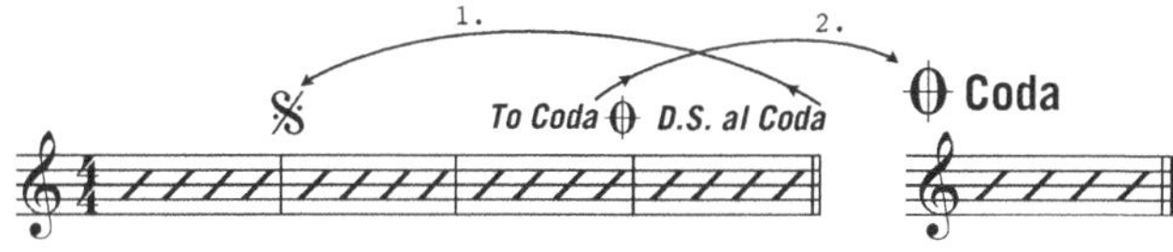

D.C. stands for *da capo* or "from the beginning." Jump to the top of the piece when you encounter this indication.

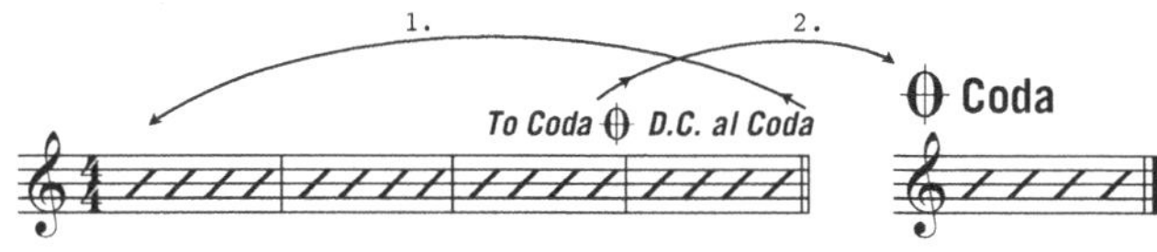

D.C. al Fine tells you to proceed to the beginning and continue until you encounter the *Fine* indicating the end of the piece (ignore the *Fine* the first time through).

CHAPTER ONE

Getting in Tune

When it comes to getting in shape, you may have experienced the saying, "The hardest part of the workout is getting to the gym." That's a very real phenomenon that musicians experience, too. Just the thought of practicing can often feel overwhelming, especially when we are confronted with thoughts such as, "I don't really know what to practice," "I'm too busy—I don't have time to get into a good practice session right now," or "There's so much to work on—where do I even begin?"

The answer is simply to start by getting into your practice space, physically and mentally, which should be a place of inspiration that welcomes creativity. Once you pick up your guitar, all those worries and judgments tend to fade away, and you can reap the rewards of playing your instrument. Some keys to successful practice sessions include clearly mapping out the things you intend to work on and for how long. This is where a practice journal can be useful. You also want to work in an environment devoid of clutter and distractions. Finally, if you have the time for a warm-up—and there's always time!—you should warm up your body with and without your guitar to reduce the risk of physical injury and fatigue.

This chapter will explore how you can organize practice materials without becoming overwhelmed, set up a functional practice space, and effectively warm up.

Prelude No. 1

Am(add9)
Am9
Em
let ring throughout

Em11
A13
A7sus2

Eadd9
F♯add9 4 / E
E6 9♯11

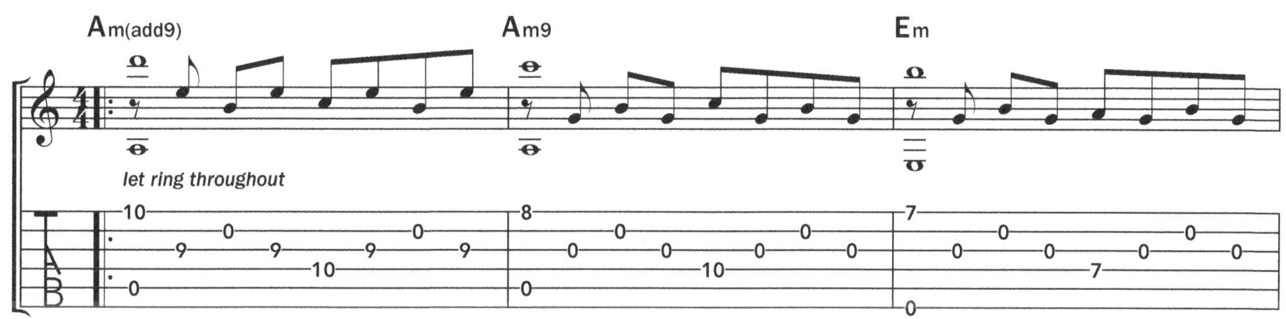

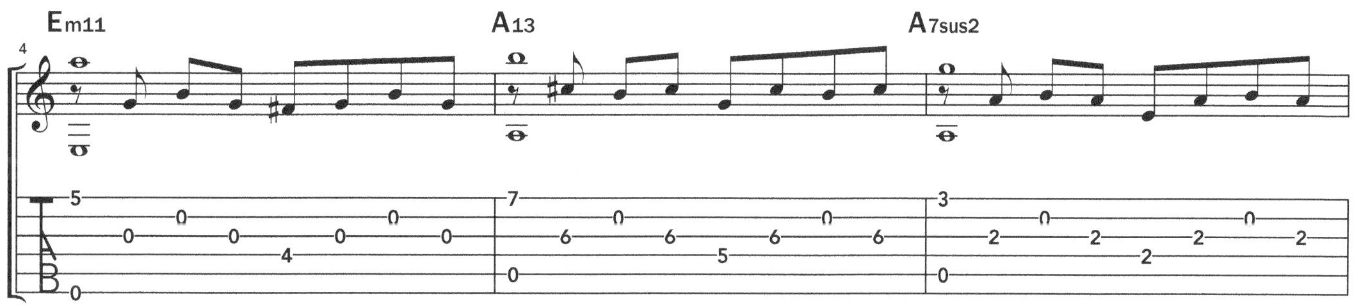

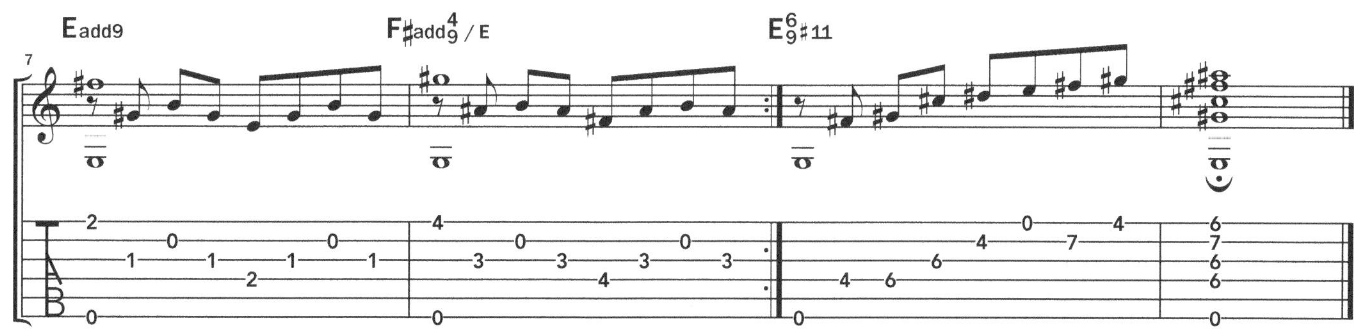

Defining Your Practice

Make a Plan

Going into a practice session, the most important strategy is simply to have a plan. Writing out your musical goals in a journal dedicated to guitar practice can help keep you focused and on task. It can also help encourage you down the road as you start to witness your own progress and development.

Quite often the content of your practice session will be determined by how much time you have, so these considerations can be planned together. The following are briefly annotated lists of four broad musical areas—musical skills and literacy, guitar technique, repertoire, and free-form—that you can draw from to organize and plan your practice time. The content within this first area of musical skills will vary depending on your own personal musical goals and professional situations, if applicable. But these topics are indeed important, as they encompass exercises in fundamentals, which even master musicians continue to work on throughout their entire career. Keep things fresh in your practice sessions by moving between topics within each area.

Musical Skills and Literacy

1 **Sight-reading**: If you are a professional guitarist, it is essential to learn to read standard notation. But even if you play casually, learning how to read will give you access to an enormously rich and rewarding library of music. While it's typically not within the culture of guitarists—compared to other string instruments—it's possible to develop sight-reading skills within a relatively short time and it is well worth the effort. The key, as with many other things, is to be consistent. It's better to practice 5–7 minutes of reading every day than a few hours occasionally.

2 **Ear-training**: This could include working with ear-training software or apps, or simply learning songs, chord progressions, and solos by ear. It will also improve your proficiency at writing music down for other musicians you play with.

3 **Music books**: Part of your session could include working with a book of concepts, songs, or guitar transcriptions by one of your favorite musicians or educators.

4 **Fretboard studies**: Learning the notes of the neck, chord shapes and voicings, scale and arpeggio patterns, voice-leading exercises, fingerings for solo lines, etc.

5 **Rhythm studies**: Developing solid time using a metronome or drum programs, playing and reading various rhythms, working on different time signatures and rhythmic styles, etc.

6 **Harmony**: Studying techniques through repertoire, analyzing chord progressions, and learning chord substitutions and reharmonization.

7 **Chord voicings**: Developing a vast vocabulary of chords and riffs to use in different styles of music and tunings, etc.

Guitar Technique

1 Picking
Developing tone, clarity, and speed using alternate picking, cross-picking, economy/directional, sweeping, hybrid, and fingerstyle techniques.

2 Fretting
Building strength, endurance, independence, and flexibility; slurs such as hammer-ons, pull-offs, and slides; string bending; pitch accuracy; articulation and touch.

3 Other techniques
Proficiency with special techniques such as harmonics, tapping, percussive effects, etc.

Repertoire

1. Learning and developing new music
2. Relearning and remembering older tunes from your repertoire
3. Expanding repertoire
4. Arranging and rearranging songs
5. Composing

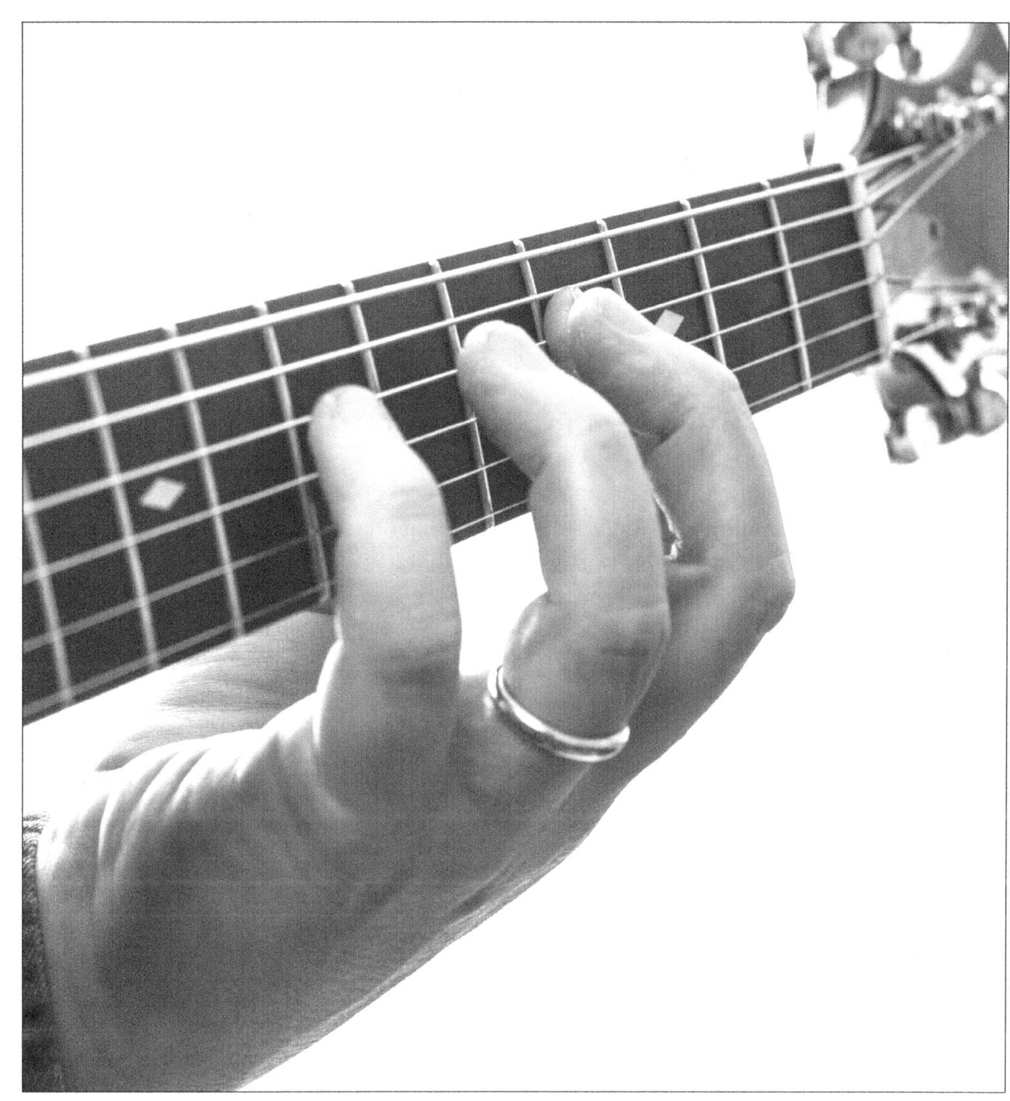

Free-Form

This area is a great way to wrap up a session by playing anything you want, having fun, and staying in a flow. Often free-form might include improvising, jamming, soloing over tracks, or developing techniques for a new song you're working on. You can also use the material you've worked on that day to create something new to play. The key word here is play.

There are several ways you can choose to structure your practice session, and this will be explored in greater detail with various practice routines in later chapters. But start by making a list of goals for the day, week, or month, and choose which area you'd like to focus on, and for how long. For example, after warming up, you could devote 15–30 minutes to one of the topics under the musical skills area (e.g., working with a book) and after a short break, allocate 20 minutes to technique, 30–45 minutes on repertoire, and close out with a free-form jam of your choice. Obviously, this will vary depending on how much time you have, but it's a good start to organizing your practice materials and goals.

Setting the Space

One of the most important considerations when establishing a solid practice routine is establishing a clean, functional, and inspiring practice space. Perhaps you have a room that you can dedicate as your studio; perhaps it's only a corner of a room in a small apartment. Regardless of the situation, your practice space should feel almost sacred in that it is exclusively devoted to creativity, growth, inspiration, and music making.

In addition to your guitar(s), consider making a list of all the tools you'll likely need in a practice session. These might include a music stand for books and sheet music, metronome, amplification, music player, audio/video recording device, notebook/journal, a timer, and any relevant accessories (e.g., capo, pencils/erasers, tuner, etc.). Many of the items on this list can be used on a computer, tablet, or smartphone; just be sure these devices aren't distracting you from practice. Avoid getting interrupted by phone calls or text messages, and refrain from using your devices for anything but music. Technology can be a useful aid, however, particularly if you are working in a smaller space. For example, a smartphone can provide a tuner, metronome, play-along apps, a clock timer, as well as music and video for reference when learning songs, and a tablet can be a great alternative to books in practice or performances, especially with a foot-controlled page turner.

Besides being functional, you also want your practice space to feel comfortable and inviting. It should be a place where you feel immediately at ease and inspired. Make sure it is well lit, with either natural or good artificial lighting that's not taxing on your eyes. Many guitarists like to add a touch of inspiration by hanging their favorite art, inspiring poetry, and/or photos of their musical heroes on the wall. Plants can also provide a nice touch to your work environment.

Make sure to keep your space relatively sparse; it should only have what you need to practice, and what inspires you. A cluttered space can tend to be off-putting and stifle productivity. Instead, strive to keep it clean, and if you'd like, rotate instruments and tools to keep things fresh.

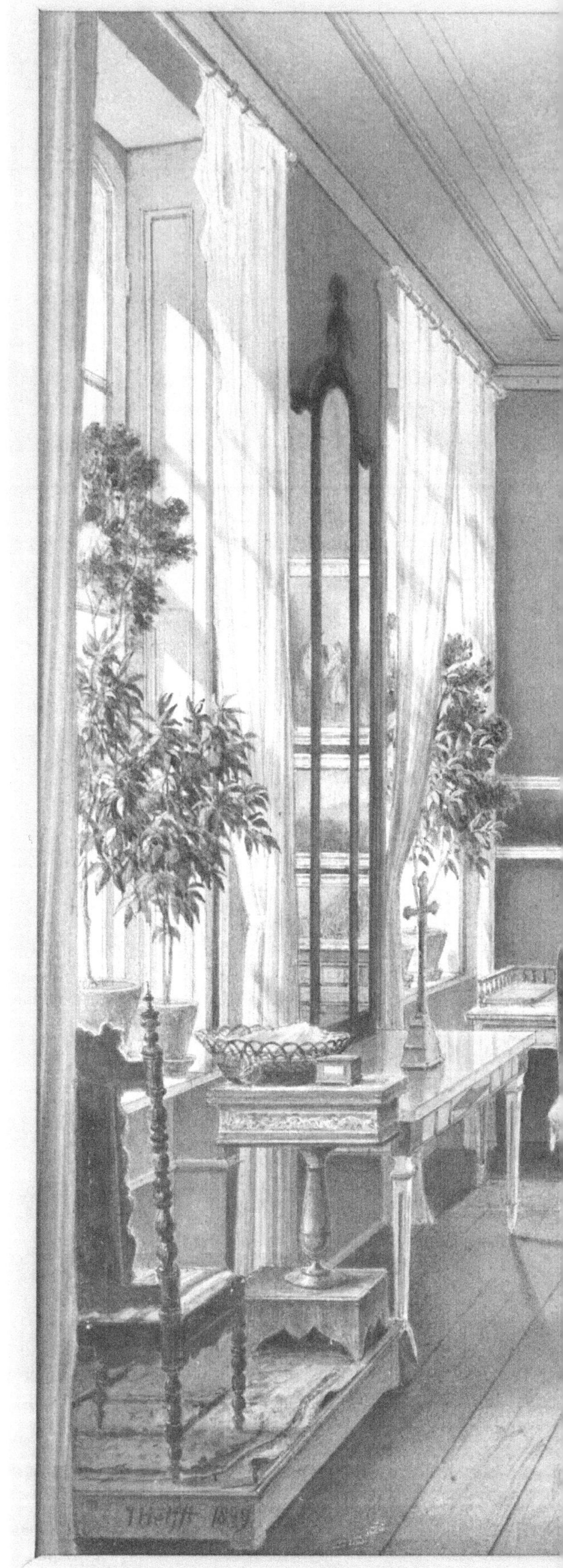

Julius Eduard Wilhelm Helfft *The Music Room of Fanny Mendelssohn*, 1849

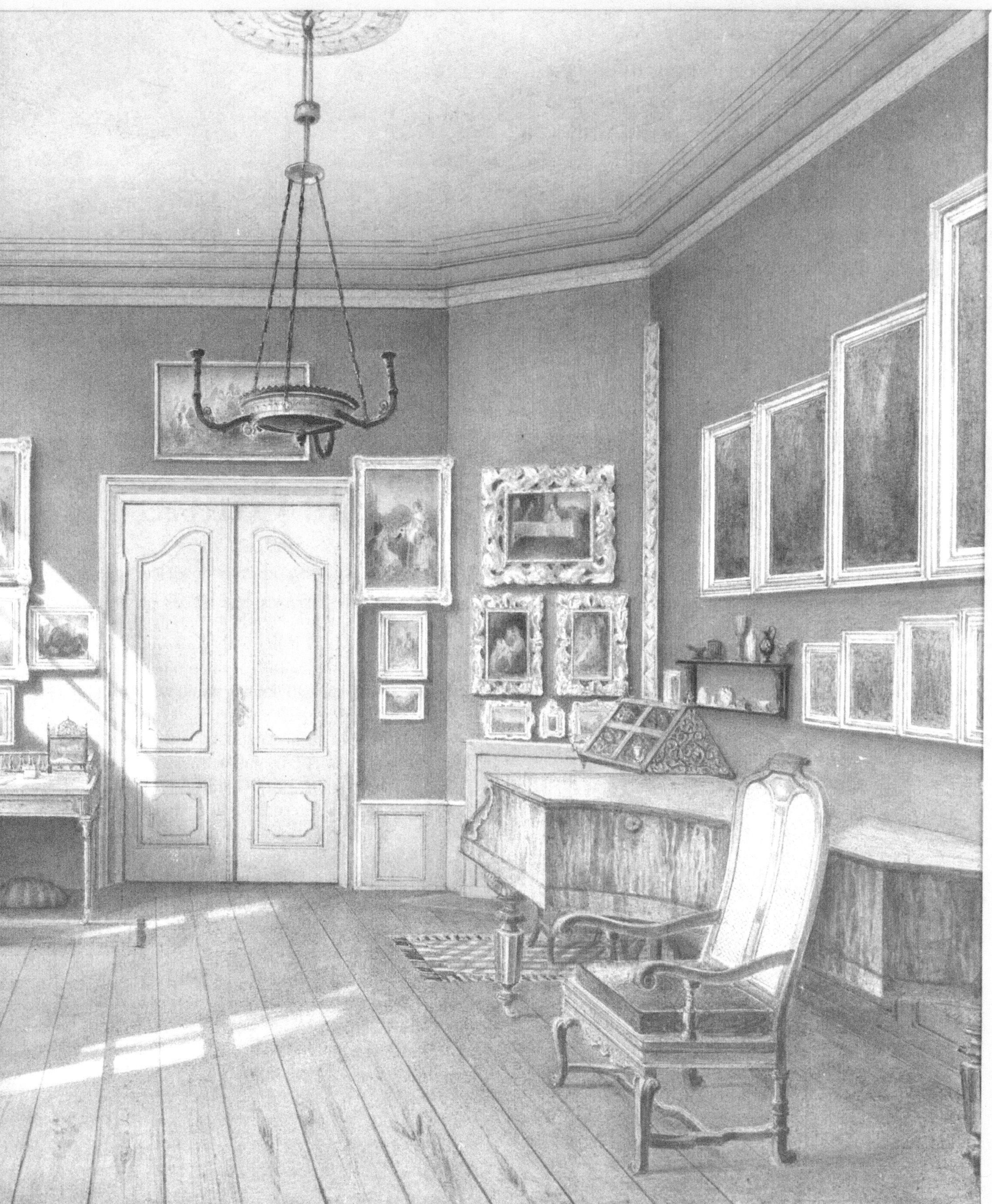

Cooper Hewitt, Smithsonian Design Museum

Ergonomics 101

The essential principle of ergonomics is a connection that results in efficiency, ease, and elegance of motion. We can apply this principle to the way we play guitar, including how we sit, stand, and hold the guitar while playing—and even the guitar itself. We also want to think about ergonomics applied to different facets of practicing and performing.

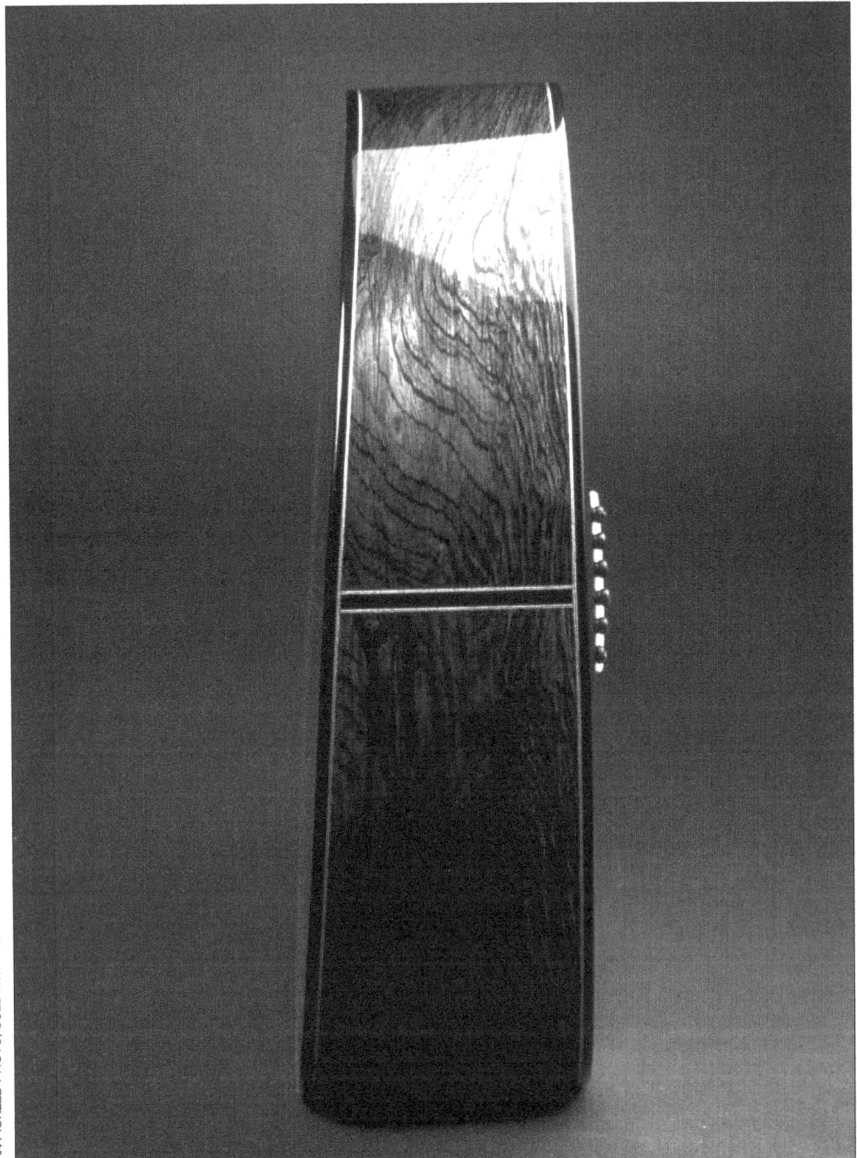

BRIAN PICKELL PHOTO, USED WITH PERMISSION

The Guitar

Many guitarists are drawn to a guitar based on its sound (and let's face it, its looks, too). But you should also notice how it feels—how it fits with your body, and how comfortable (or uncomfortable) is it to play. Obviously, you'll want to do things like get it set up properly and find the right string gauges, but also consider the depth of the guitar, the shape of the body, and the width of the lower bout, all of which determine how it fits with your body type, arm length, and hand size. You can also consider scale length and nut width based on your physical size, as well as your style of playing. The Linda Manzer wedge is one example of the way contemporary luthiers and manufacturers are building acoustic and archtop guitars with ergonomic designs that include arm bevels, fanned frets, and tapered bodies.

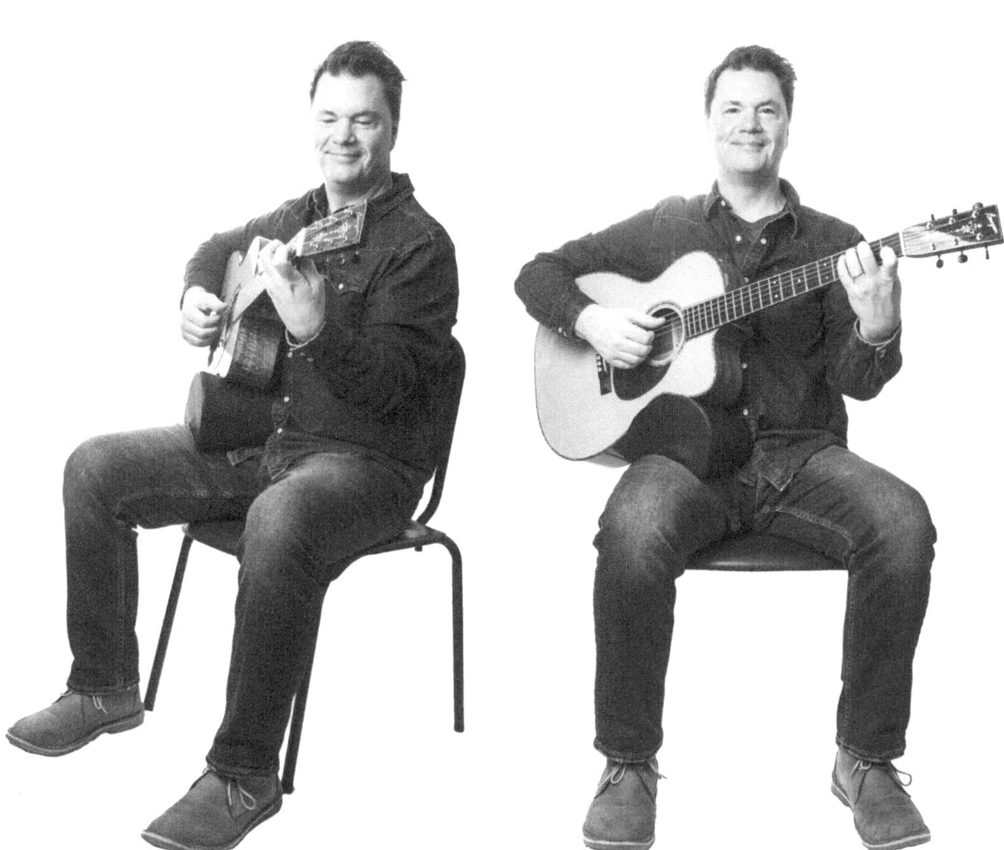

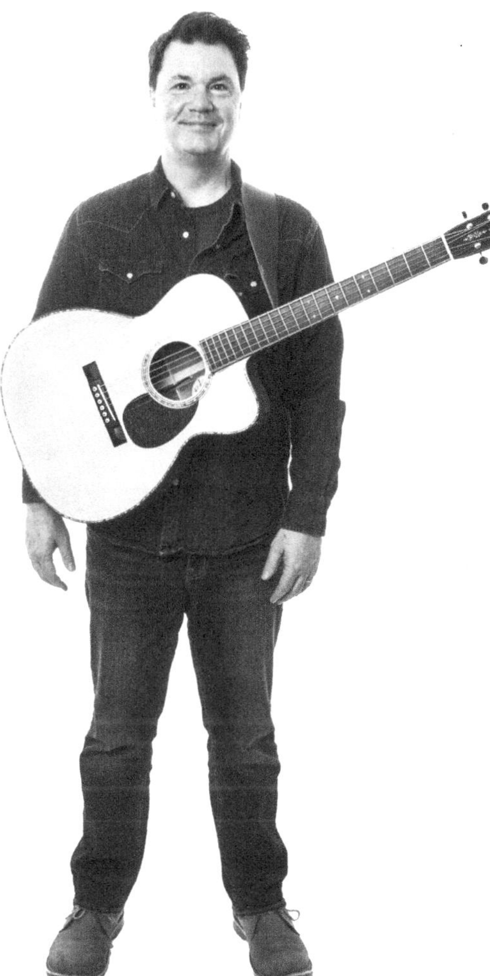

Sitting with the Guitar

When studying classical instruments, quite often the first thing students learn is how to sit and/or stand with their instruments, which is in direct contrast to most self-taught players and/or pop-rock oriented guitarists. It might seem obvious, but learning and practicing how to sit with the guitar effortlessly is an important element to remaining injury-free while practicing and performing for long hours at a time.

Start by using an armless chair or stool that is comfortable. Both of your feet should be planted flat on the floor with the guitar resting gently in your lap. Try to avoid using a footstool or propping one leg up higher than the other, as this creates an asymmetrical imbalance in the hips and lower back that can lead to problems over time. If you need to elevate your guitar to maintain a correct and comfortable posture (typically, the guitar neck will be roughly at a 45-degree angle to facilitate easy access to the entire fretboard), try using a cushion balanced on either the right or left leg. Many contemporary players prefer to use devices such as a cushion or tripod that rests on the leg with suction cups that affix to the back of the guitar, allowing it to be played at a higher level. The legendary fingerstyle guitarist Pierre Bensusan, for example, is a longtime user of one such product, the NeckUp guitar support.

Try sitting in your chair without a guitar, relaxed but with a straight spine, your feet on the floor in front of you. Keep your hips pointed slightly forward, with your spine comfortably in an upward position. You'll notice that if you roll your hips back, you'll be in a common slouching position. Instead, gently roll your hips forward, and you'll feel your spine straightening and elongating. Now get into a guitar-playing position. Your fretting hand should be at a comfortable level just under your shoulder, and your picking hand should be resting around your midsection, as if you naturally dropped your arm into your body. This is how you want to feel and look with (and without) your guitar.

Standing with the Guitar

I recommend using a wide (2-1/2- to 3-1/2-inch) strap with good padding whether you are sitting or standing. If you are standing, your strap should support your guitar without pinching your neck or shoulder, and a good strap will allow you to play at the same angle when you're sitting. Make sure you put equal weight on each leg to support the guitar with your core while your shoulders and upper back are relaxed.

Warming Up the Body

It's certainly tempting to pick up the guitar and start playing cold, and it's fine to do that from time to time, especially on occasions when you're inspired. But it's better to start with a brief body warm-up and stretching session as a prelude to a practice session. Here is a list of stretches and easy-to-do exercises that will prime your body to get in a good practice state and reduce the chances of repetitive use injuries. Feel free to do all or mix it up with just a few of these every day. These exercises will only take a few minutes and they'll help your body feel strong and relaxed. Before you know it, these become a welcome habit to your daily routine.

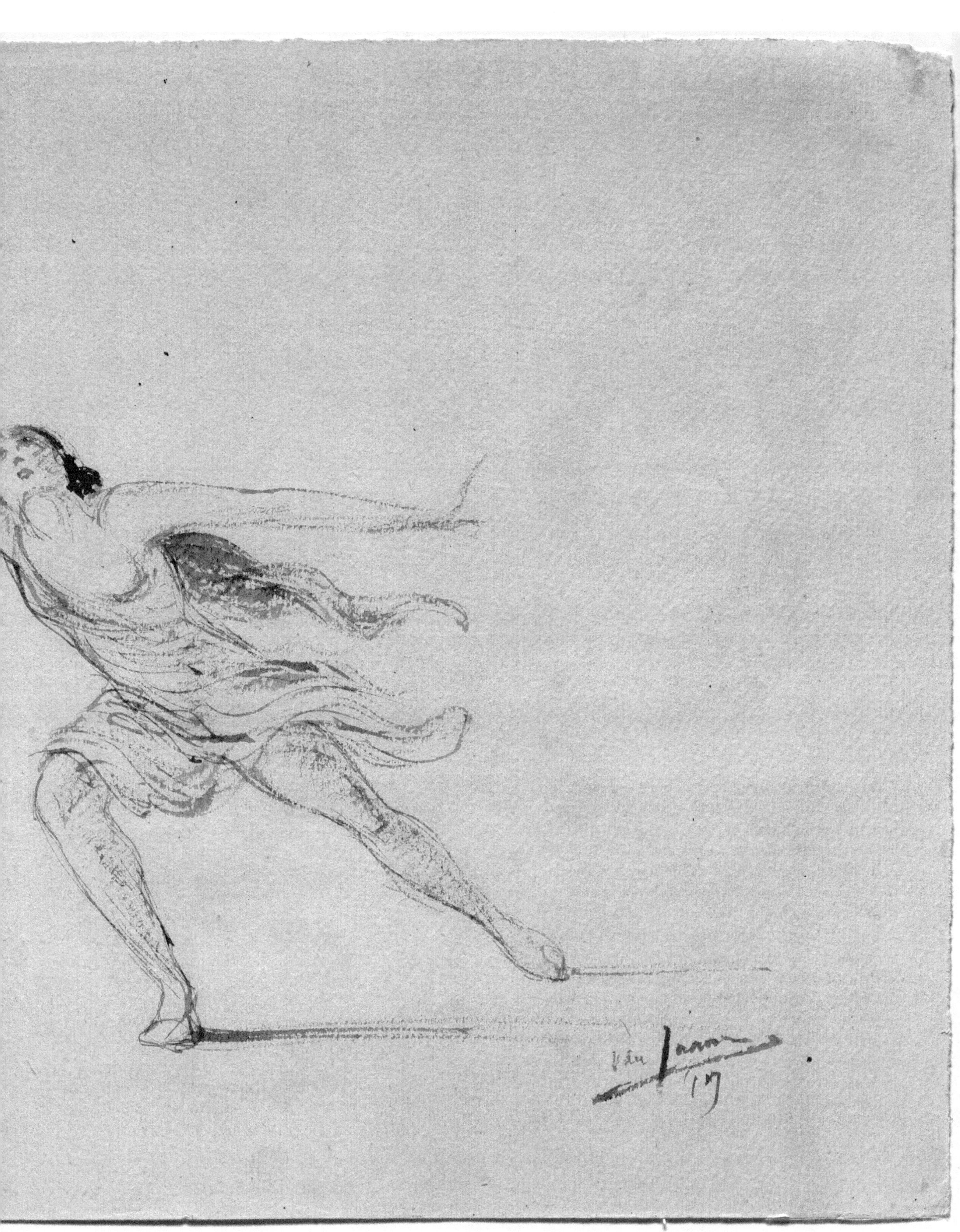

Basic Stretches

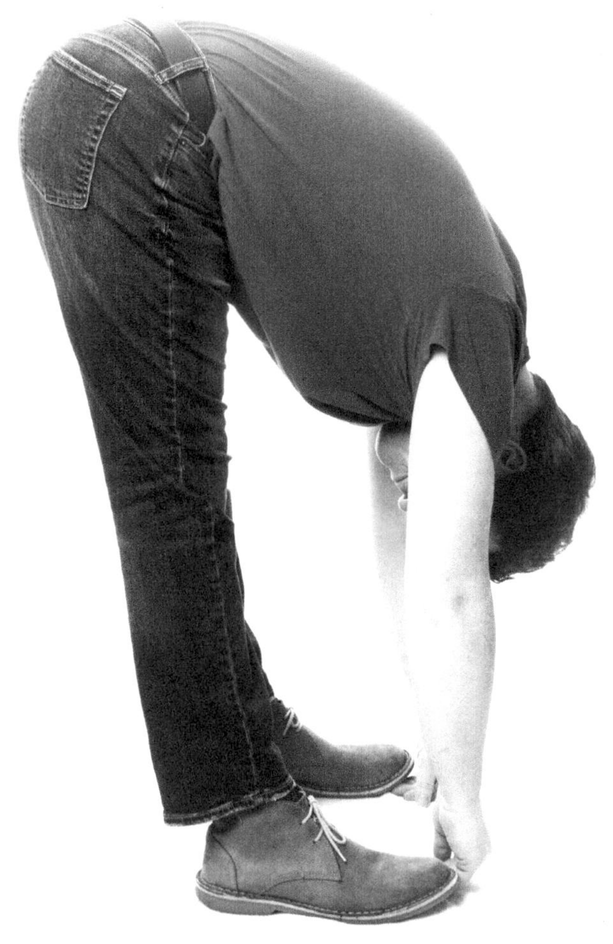

1. Backside/hamstring stretch: Stand up straight and relax into a shoulder-width stance, finding your balance and taking two or three deep breaths, inhaling into the abdomen, and exhaling slowly. Stretch both arms straight up above your body and slowly bend forward to touch the floor, your feet, or ankles, or as far is comfortable. Remember to breathe while slowly lowering your torso. Hold this posture for a few seconds and notice a stretch in the back of your legs, calves, and spine. Slowly return your upper body up to standing position, unfurling your spine one vertebrae at a time while exhaling. Try to imagine leaning up against a sturdy brick wall to support you and keep your legs and back straight as you return to starting position. Repeat two or three times.

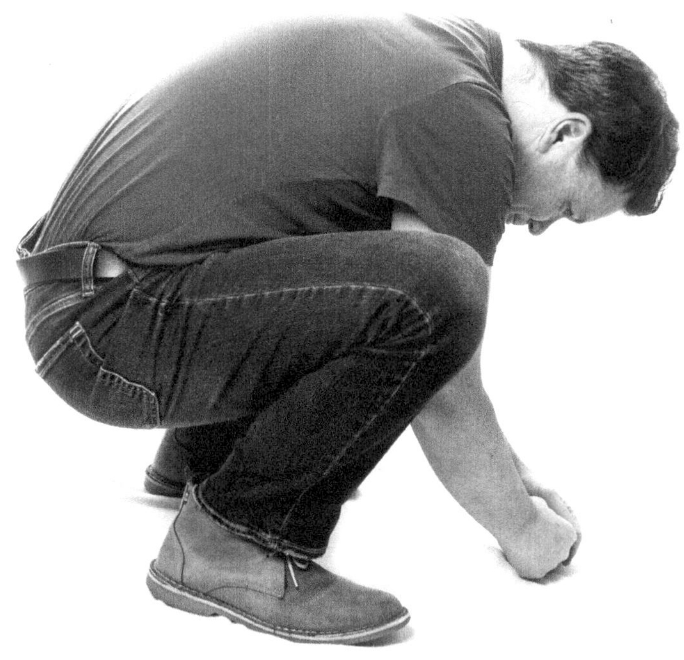

Variation: Instead of keeping your legs straight and knees softly locked, bend your knees all the way down to the floor so that you're in a crouching position with your torso in between each of your legs. Breathe deeply, straighten your legs, and slowly unfurl your back to starting position.

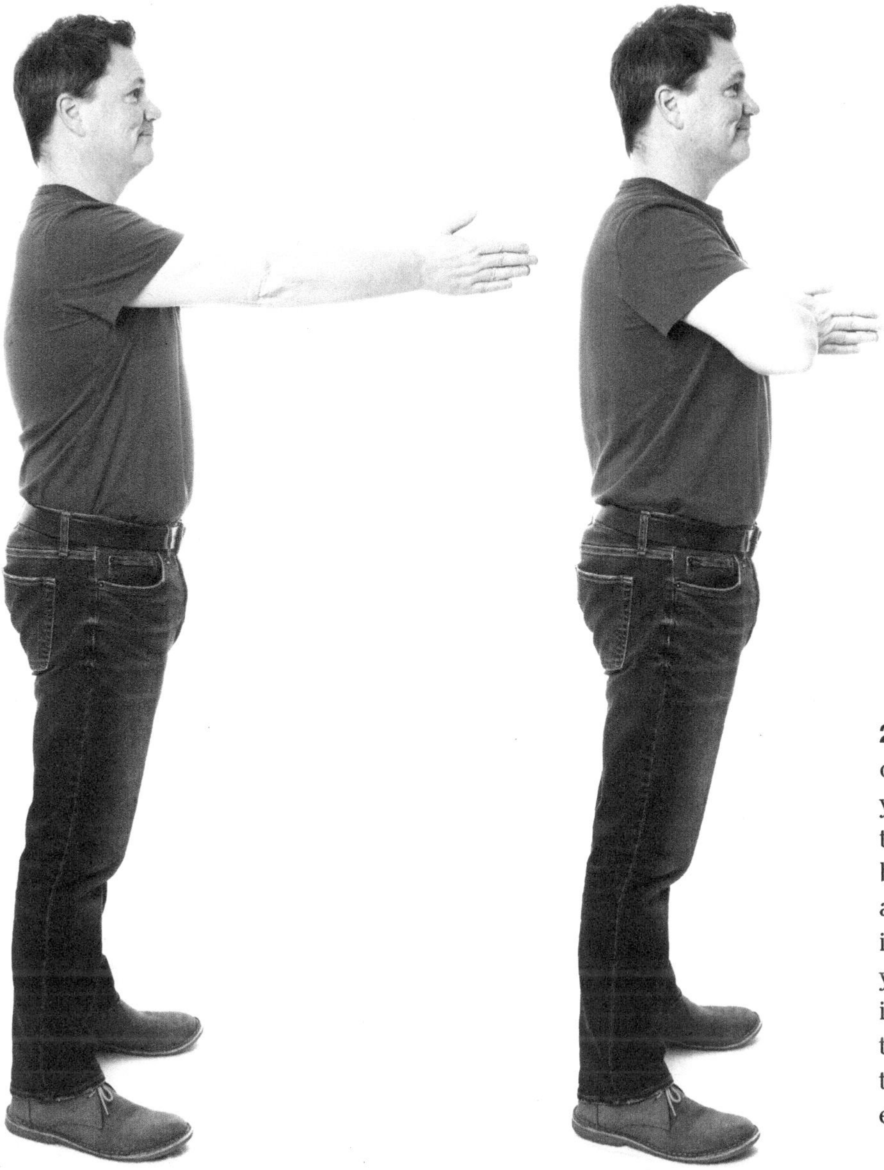

2. Wrist stretch: Hold both arms out straight in front of you with your palms facing each other and touching. Take a deep breath, slowly bring your arms into your chest, and bend your elbows while keeping your palms held together until you reach your chest (or as far as is comfortable). Hold for two to three seconds, then gradually bring the arms to starting position while exhaling.

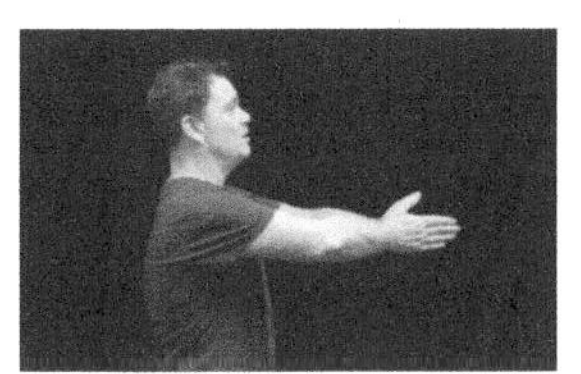

Video Resource

Watch Sean perform these stretches

3. Finger stretch: Gently but assertively stretch the fingers of each hand, one at a time, side to side and back and forth. Be careful not to overstretch any of the fingers—it should feel good and make your hands feel more pliable. It's a good idea to run your hands under warm water and then stretch them out to get the blood circulating, especially if you live in a climate with dry, cold temperatures.

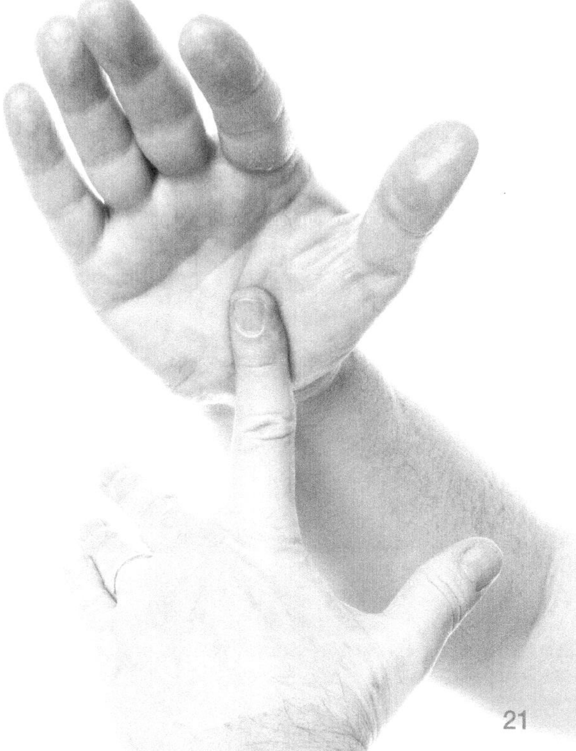

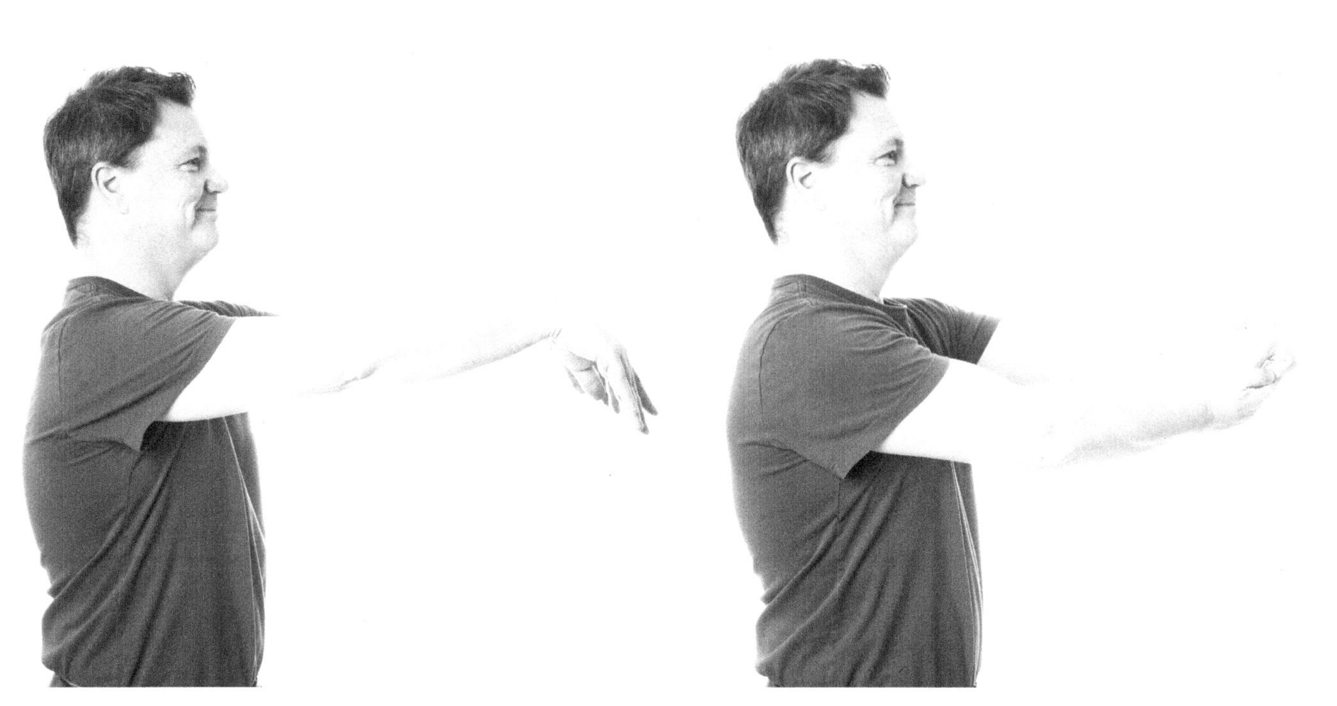

4. Forearm stretch: Stand with your arms out in front of you, elbows pointed to the floor, wrists and hands dangling freely. Take your right hand, reach over to the top of the left hand, and gently push the top of the left hand inward while rotating your left elbow back and forth, as if your elbow was a swinging hinge and drawing a small arc side to side. Repeat with the other hand and arm.

Variation: Return to starting position, but this time, face your palms forward as if you're telling someone to stop. With your right hand, very gently push the tops of the fingers of the left hand toward your body, feeling a stretch on the underside of the ulna (forearm). Repeat with the other side.

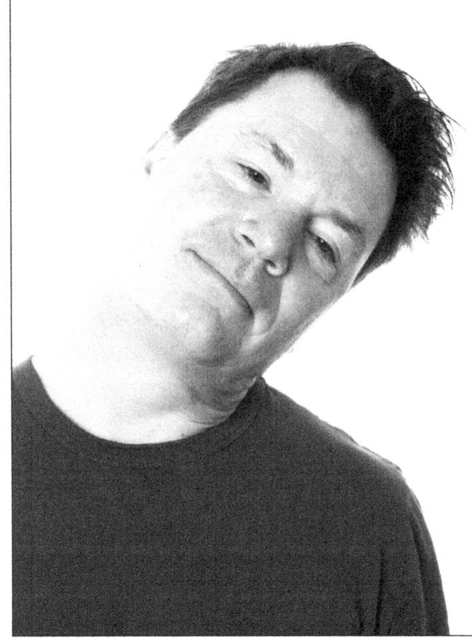

5. Neck stretch: Stand up straight with your arms relaxed on both sides of your body. Slowly stretch your neck to the right as if you're trying to connect your right ear to your shoulder. While doing this, lower your left shoulder towards the floor. You should feel a significant stretch on your left side, as this will open your neck and shoulders, which often get cramped or unbalanced while playing guitar. Repeat with the opposite side.

6. Doorway chest and arm stretch: Find a doorway slightly wider than your body. Using the doorway for support, place each of your palms flat against the doorframe at about neck level, and allow your body to slowly fall forward, keeping both feet in place and your back straight. You'll feel a solid stretch in both sides of the chest and both arms on the inside. Lean forward as far as what's comfortable and gradually come back to starting position. Wait 10–15 seconds and then raise your palms up higher to ear level. Repeat the same stretch by gently and slowly leaning forward, letting the doorway prevent you from falling forward.

Basic Warm-Up Exercises

1. Alternating knee raise: Raise both of your hands, palms facing forward, to neck height just above each shoulder. Hold while raising one knee and then the other up to your chest. Aim the right knee up toward the left chest and vice versa, alternating breathwork (five times each side).

2. Waist side bends and rotation circles: Keeping your back straight, hold on to your waist with both hands and gently bend, alternating to each side while breathing evenly (three to five times each side). Now gently move your waist in a circular movement, first clockwise and then counterclockwise, three to five times each side.

3. Arms in the air circles: Hold your arms straight out to each side, perpendicular to your body. Create circles in the air by moving your arms clockwise and counterclockwise. You can alternate between small, rapid circles and slower, larger ones (five times each direction).

4. Folding arm scissors: Once you return to starting position with the previous exercise, bring each hand in to meet the shoulders, bending at the elbow and creating a scissor-like motion while the upper arm stays static and held in place (five to 10 times, both arms folding in at the same time). Then, with your arms held straight out to the side, imagine you are opening doors with each hand keeping both arms extended and straight, perpendicular to your body, while gently rotating both wrists in a circular motion, as if they were turning a doorknob in the air (five times).

5. Shoulder wheel shrugs: Return to original standing position and shrug both of your shoulders, moving in a wheel-like motion around your ears in both directions (five times each, forward and backward).

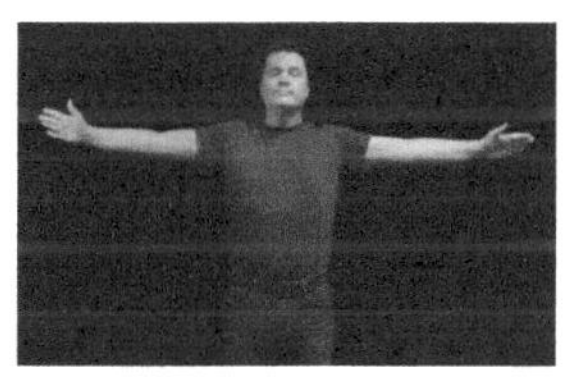

Video Resource

Watch Sean perform these stretches

The Guitar

Warming Up the Hands and Waking Up the Mind

After you've warmed up your body, it's a good idea to start slowly once you pick up the guitar, especially if it's been a few days since you last played. Our goal is to warm up the brain and ears, as well as the hands. This way, you make the best use of your time, incorporating several concepts into one exercise. We'll explore this further in later chapters on creative practicing.

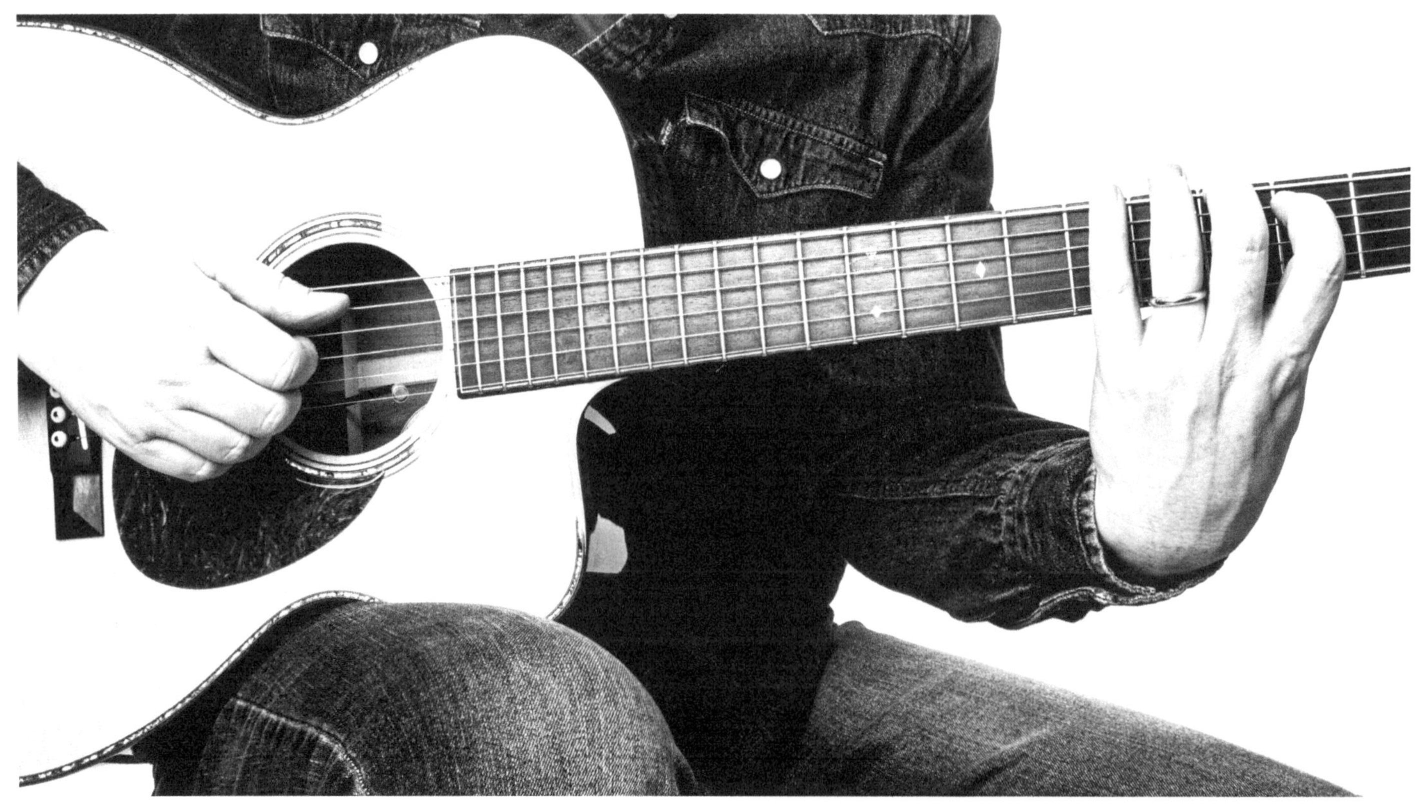

Let's begin by putting our hands on the strings. **Example 1** is a simple exercise for basic synchronization with both hands. These first few examples are similar to time-honored classical guitar exercises used to wake up the hands and feel the strings. We can also use these examples to train our ears and work on basic theory exercises. **Example 2** threads a melodic line that connects diatonic chords in the key of G major. We can also explore inner lines and basic voice-leading through a progression while warming up, as shown in **Examples 3** and **4**.

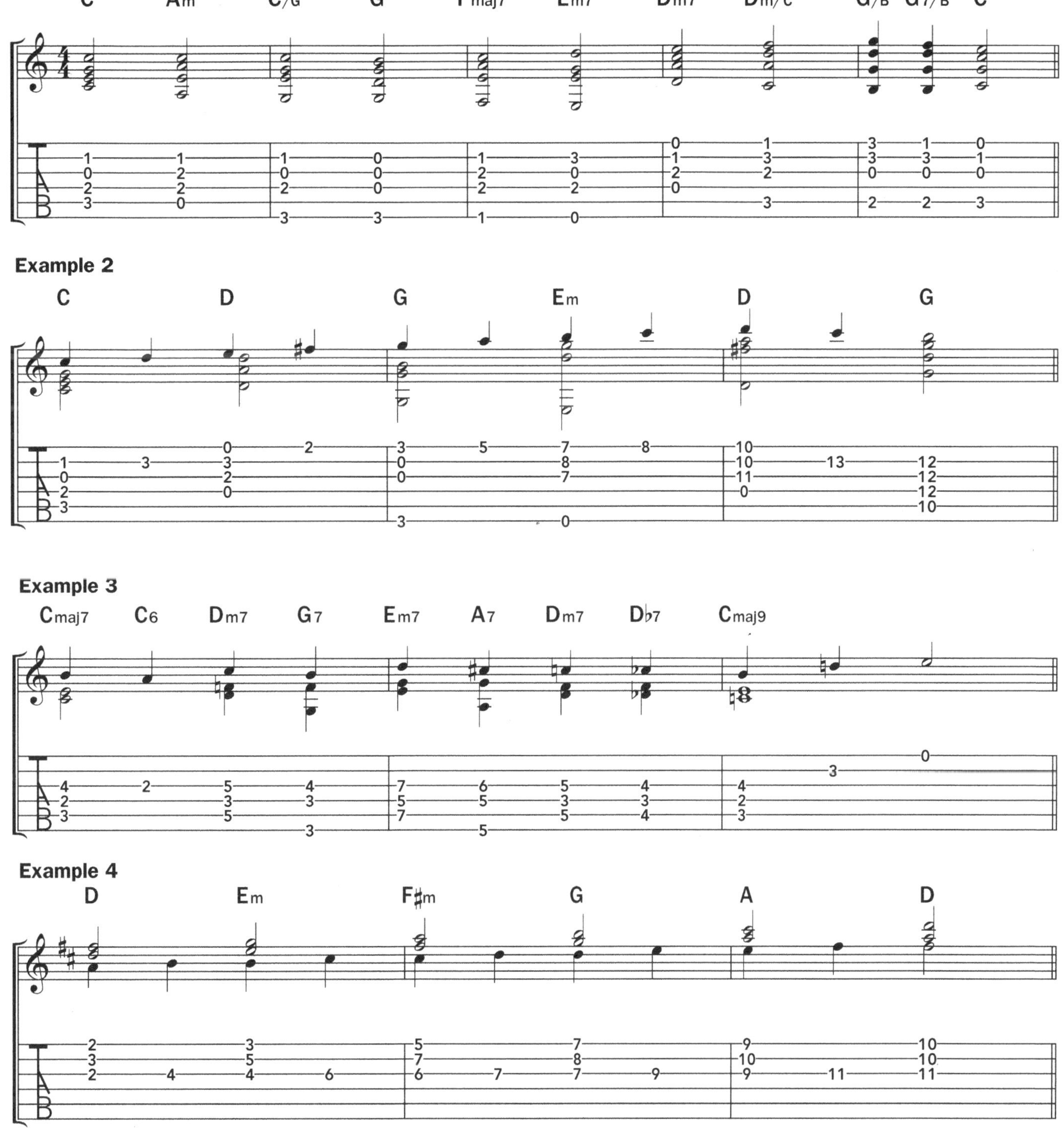

Example 5 illustrates a comprehensive triad voice-leading exercise using a I–IV–V–I (A–D–E–A) progression in the key of A major, which is also an effective switching exercise for the fingers of the fretting hand. These are like basic piano exercises, simultaneously developing finger coordination, knowledge of voice-leading, and the ability to hear basic harmonic structures.

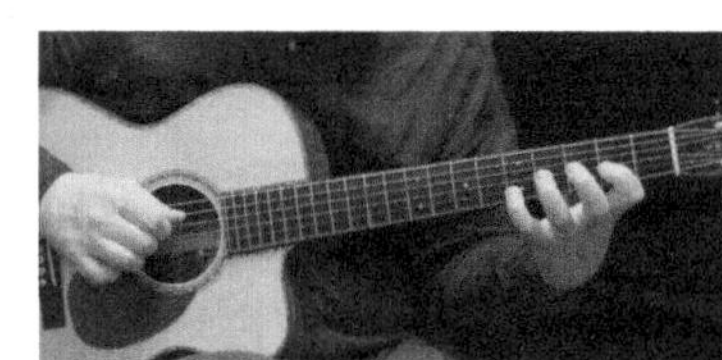

Video Resource

Watch Sean play through these examples

Example 5

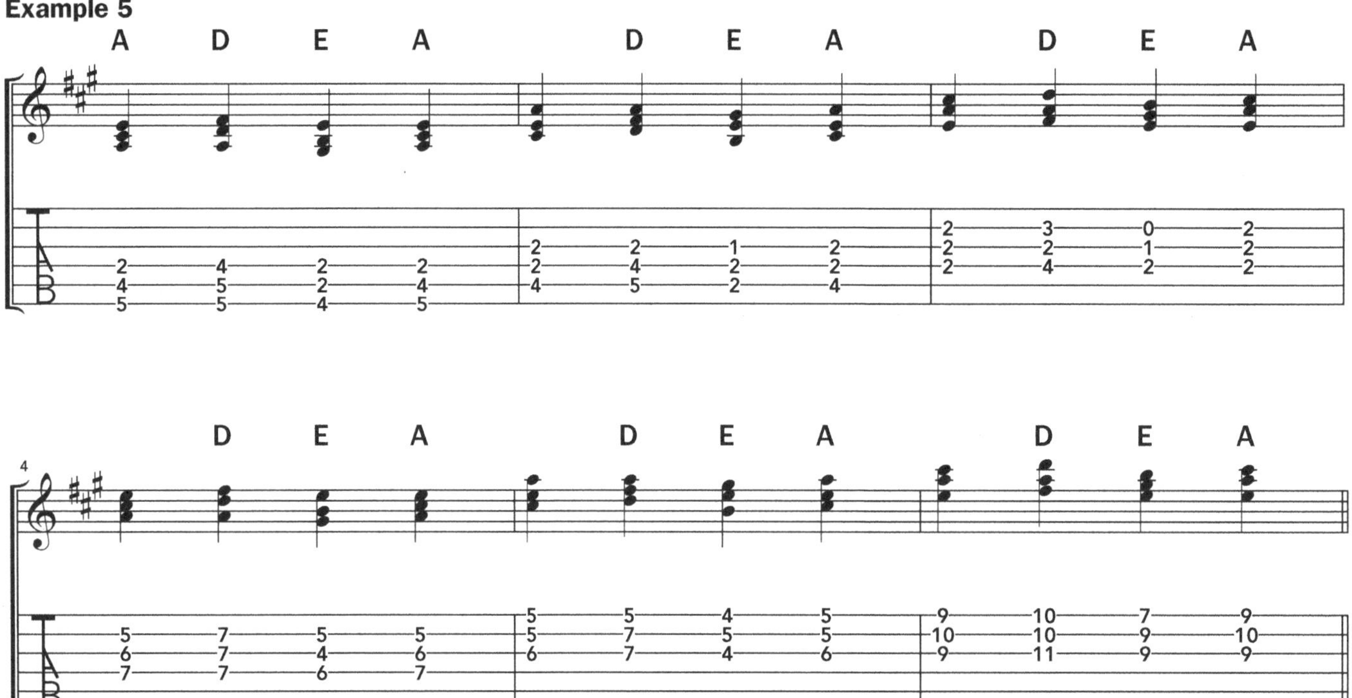

Examples 6a–b move triad inversions of G major and minor across all string sets and provide an excellent warm-up for the picking hand, whether you play with a pick or fingerstyle. As your hands begin to warm up, you can increase the difficulty a notch by playing expansive G major and minor arpeggios in triplets (**Examples 7a–b**). Of course, you can substitute any root or arpeggio type as these are all movable forms.

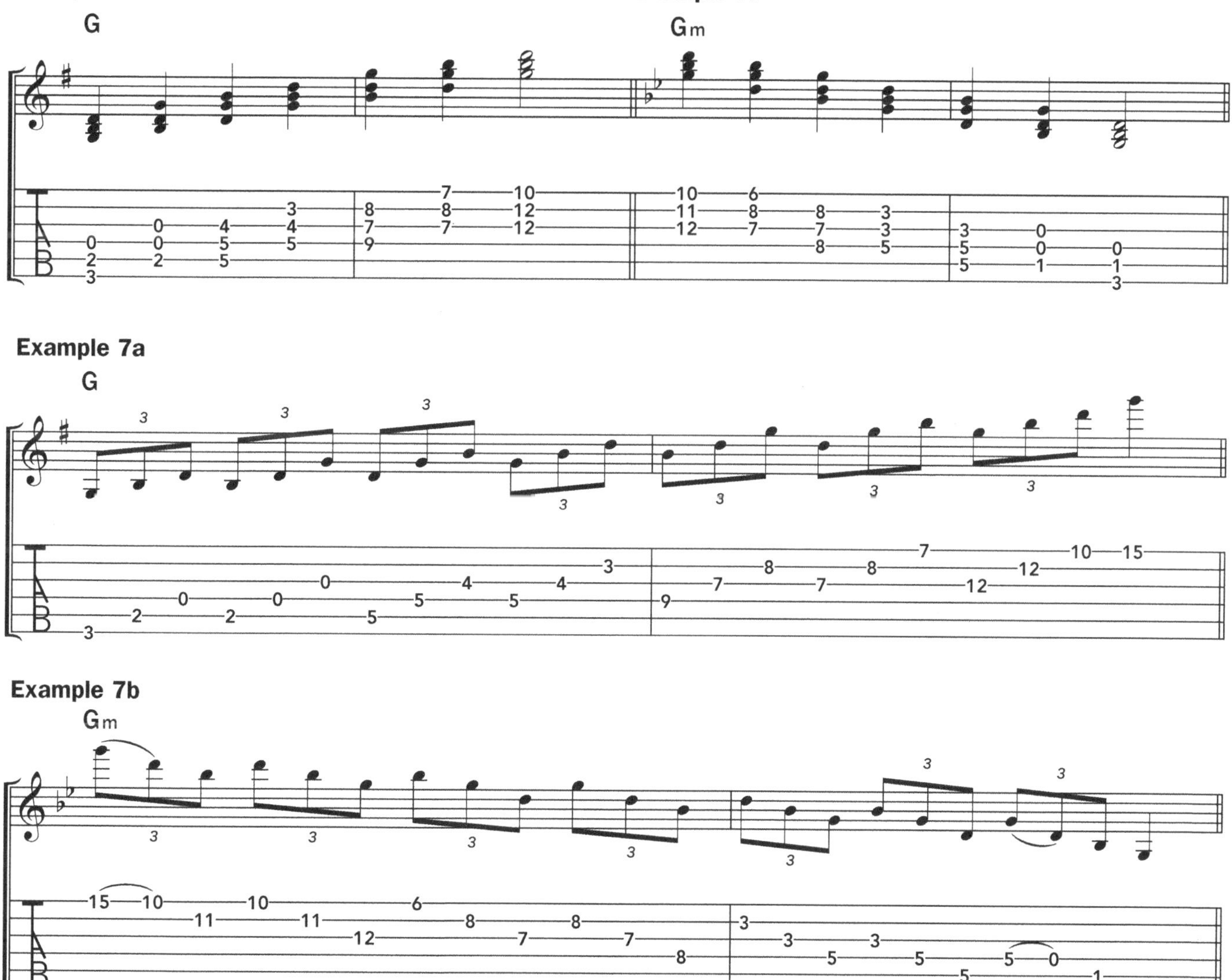

You may have noticed by now that the warm-up didn't begin with scales. For good reason—these come later, as we don't want to start with too rigorous an exercise. Now that you've acclimated your body and hands to the instrument, you can work on some scale patterns as shown in **Examples 8a–c**, which showcase major, Dorian/minor, and dominant scales ascending in double-stops before descending as a single line in different rhythms.

Examples 9a–c explore challenging string crossing exercises for both hands, exploring ninth patterns for major, minor, and dominant chord types. Be sure to take these sets of exercises slowly, preferably with a metronome; always strive for clarity, accuracy, and good tone.

Our warm-up concludes with some basic grooves that are fun to play. In **Examples 10a–b**, we have examples of a 1970s funk groove with an E9 chord, and a flatpicking riff using open strings, slides, and hammer-ons. If you're running short on time, you don't necessarily need to play these examples in their entirety, but it is imperative to start out slowly and simply, gradually working your way through the various techniques before starting your practice session or performance.

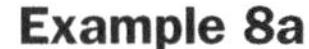

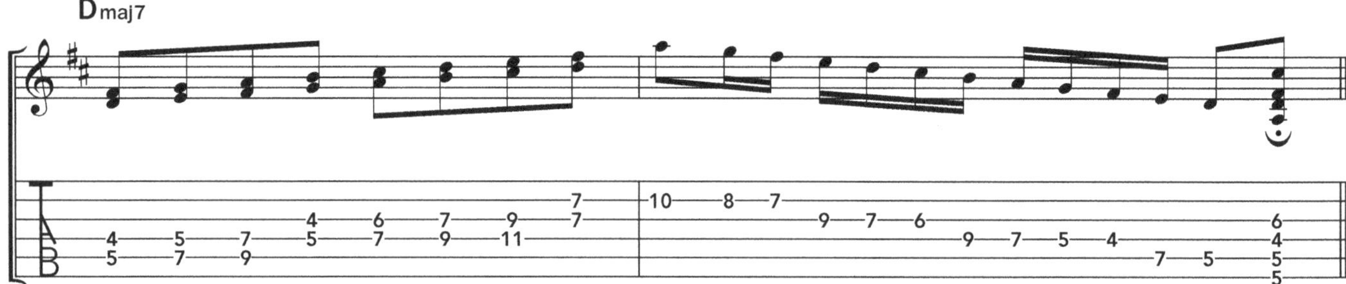

Example 8b

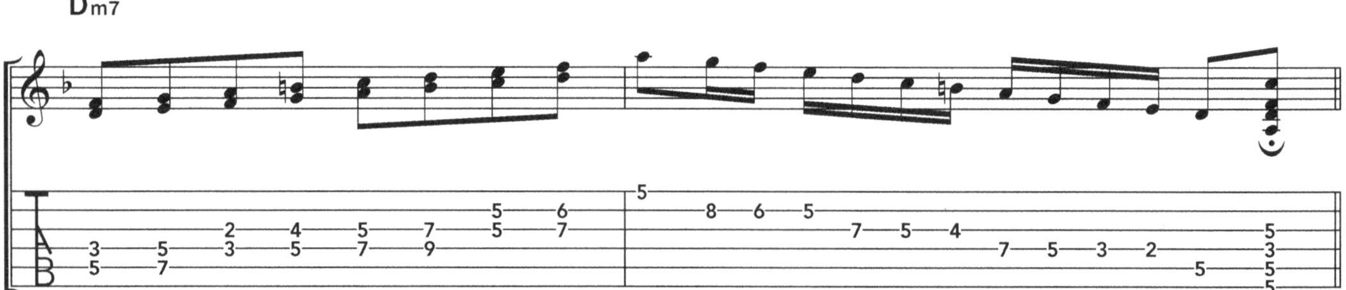

Example 8c

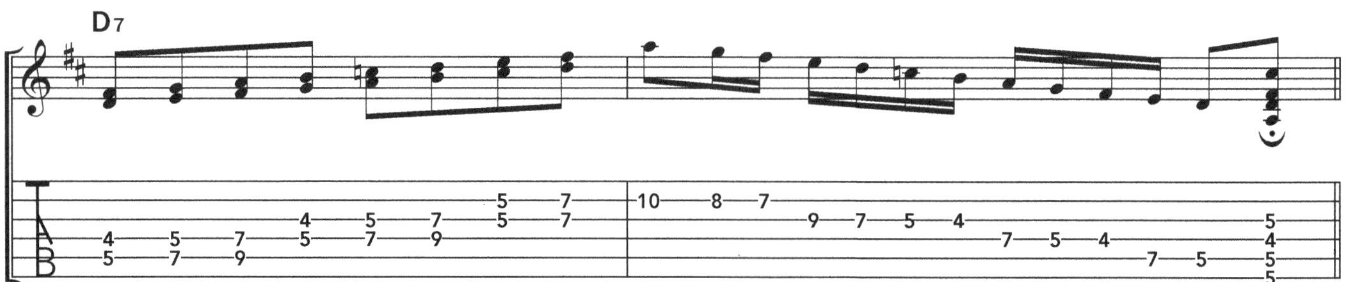

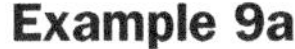

Example 9a

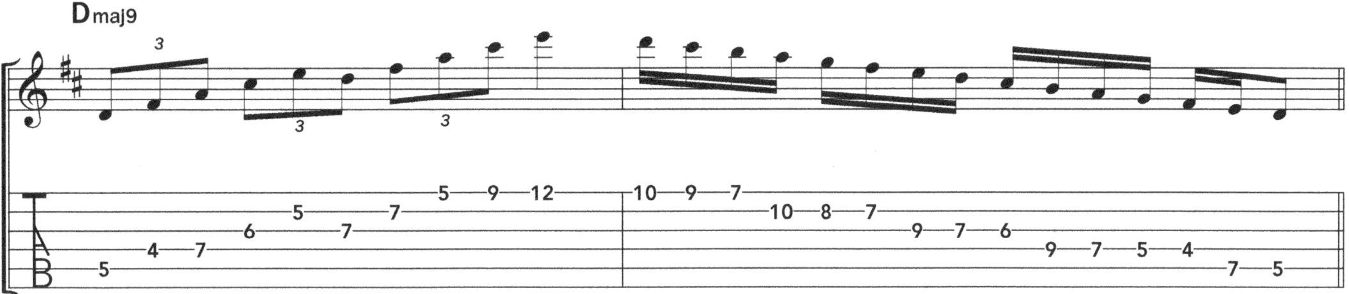

Example 9b

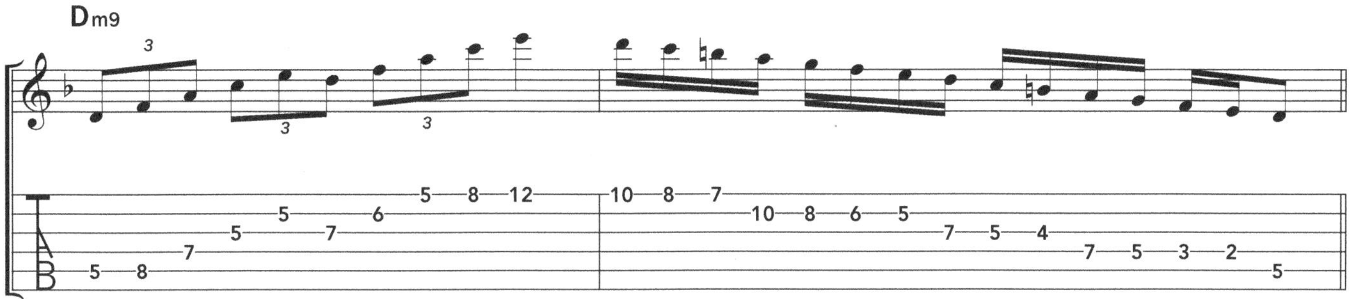

Example 9c

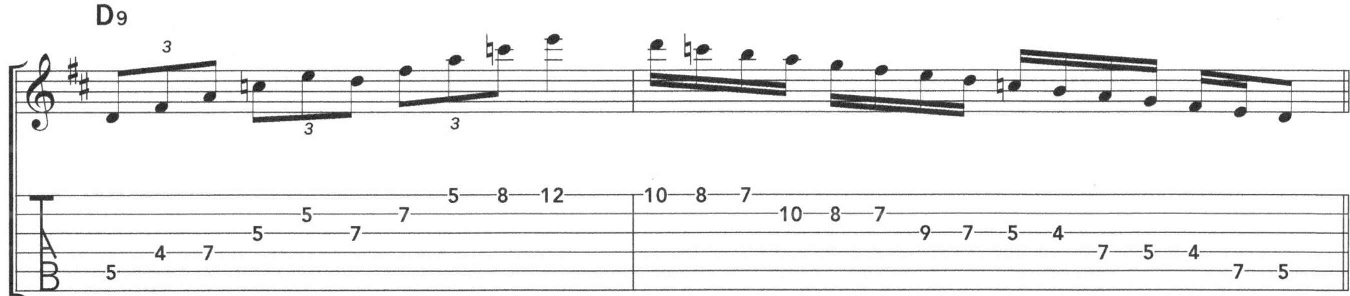

Example 10a

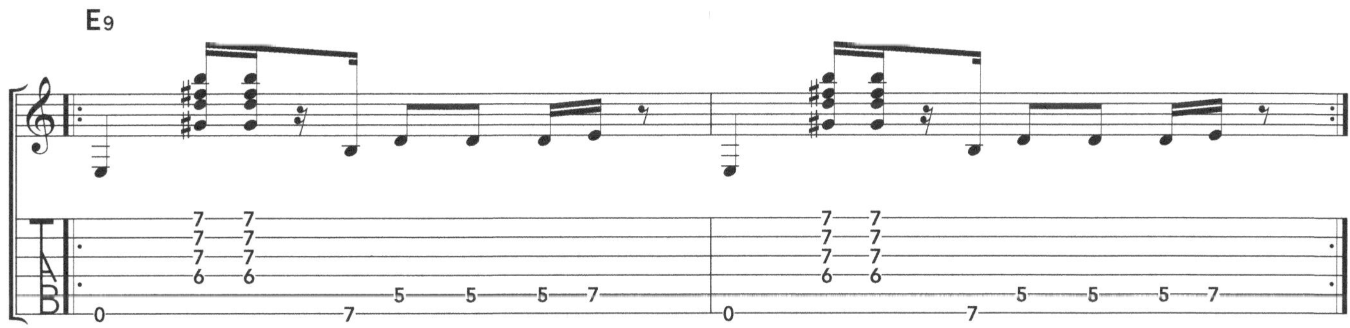

Example 10b

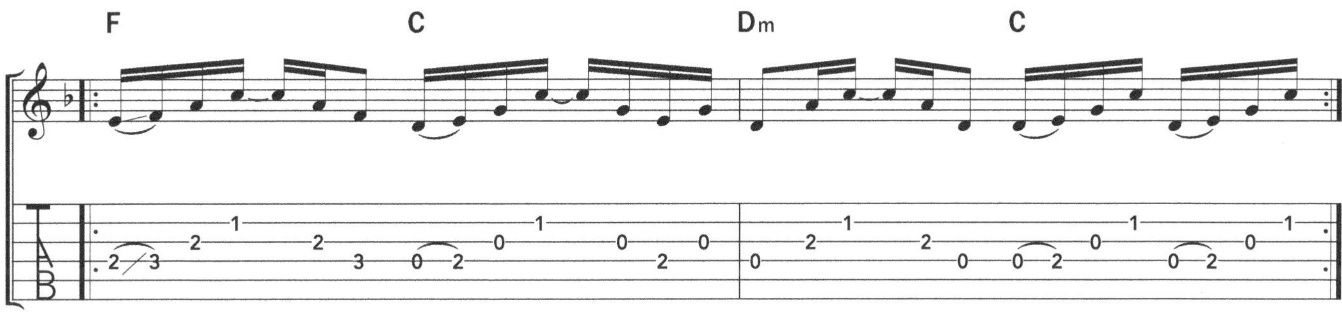

CHAPTER TWO

An Overview of Common Injuries Among Guitarists

One of the deepest tragedies to befall any musician is losing the ability to play their instrument. Playing the guitar requires significant attention to the fingers, hands, wrists, shoulders, back—indeed, the entire body. Guitarists don't tend to think of themselves as athletes, but the truth is that they must be careful to avoid the idiosyncratic injuries that can afflict them through cumulative trauma, excessive repetition, tension, poor posture, and non-musical activities (NMAs). All guitarists—regardless of age, style, or ability—benefit by knowing preventative approaches, as well as resources for healing should they experience any type of injury, whether musculoskeletal (back, neck, shoulder, arthritic pain, etc.) or musculotendinous (related to muscular and tendinous tissue).

Hearing health, especially the prevention of hearing loss and tinnitus, is also a big part of general physical wellness for musicians. This chapter will outline and define the most common injuries that tend to affect guitarists. Unfortunately, many bad habits cultivated—and ignored—in practice and performance can gradually lead to pain or injury. Fortunately, the body is responsive and will often provide signs or warnings, from mild to more severe pain or burning sensations, numbness, aching, and/or sensations in the nerves and muscles throughout the upper body. To avoid these types of injuries, the first step is to understand some basic anatomy and to create an acute self-awareness of posture, ergonomics, and energy exertion while playing the guitar.

Prelude No. 2

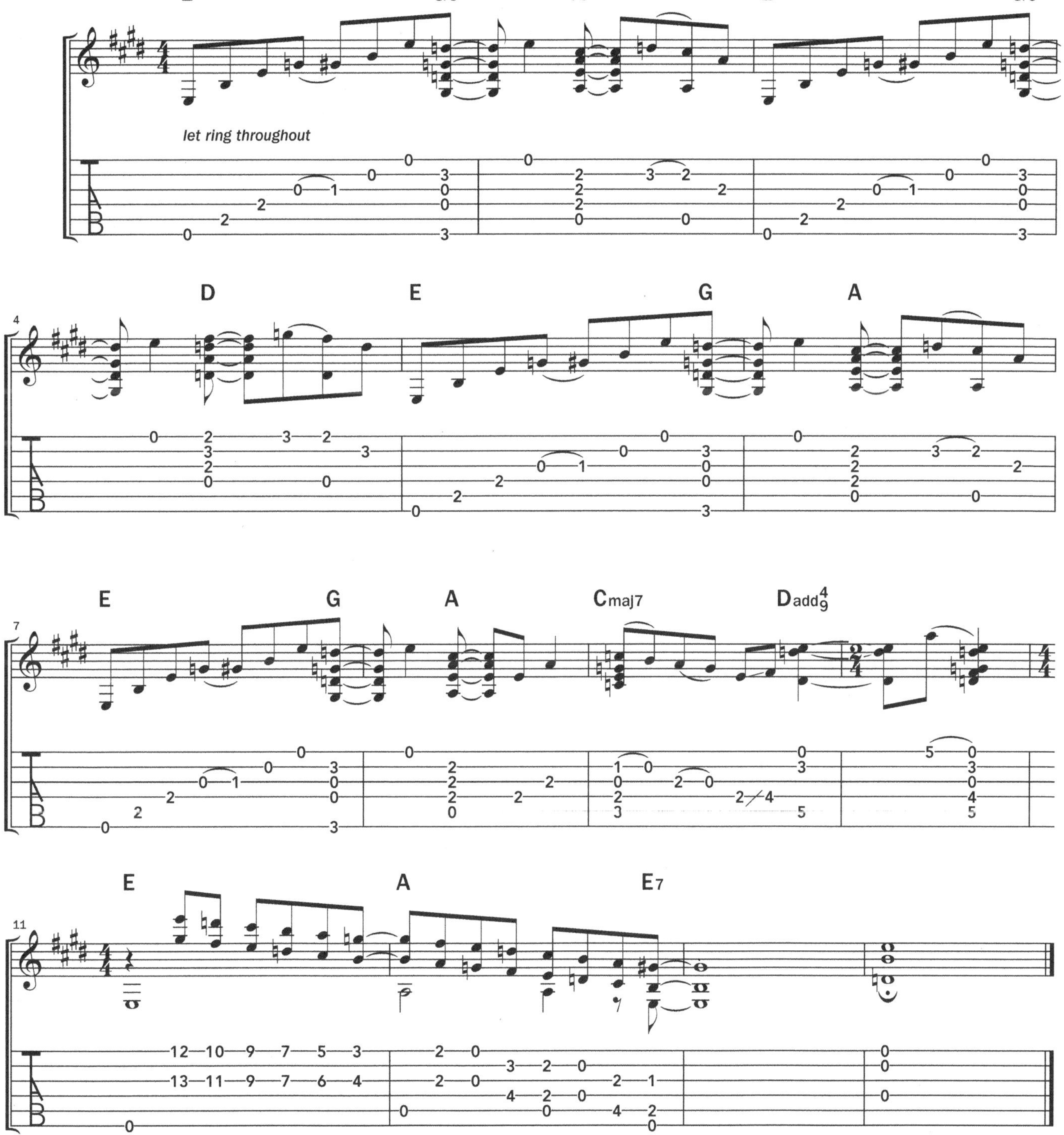

Repetitive Motion and Cumulative Trauma Syndromes in the Hands and Wrists

Tendonitis *(Tendinitis)*

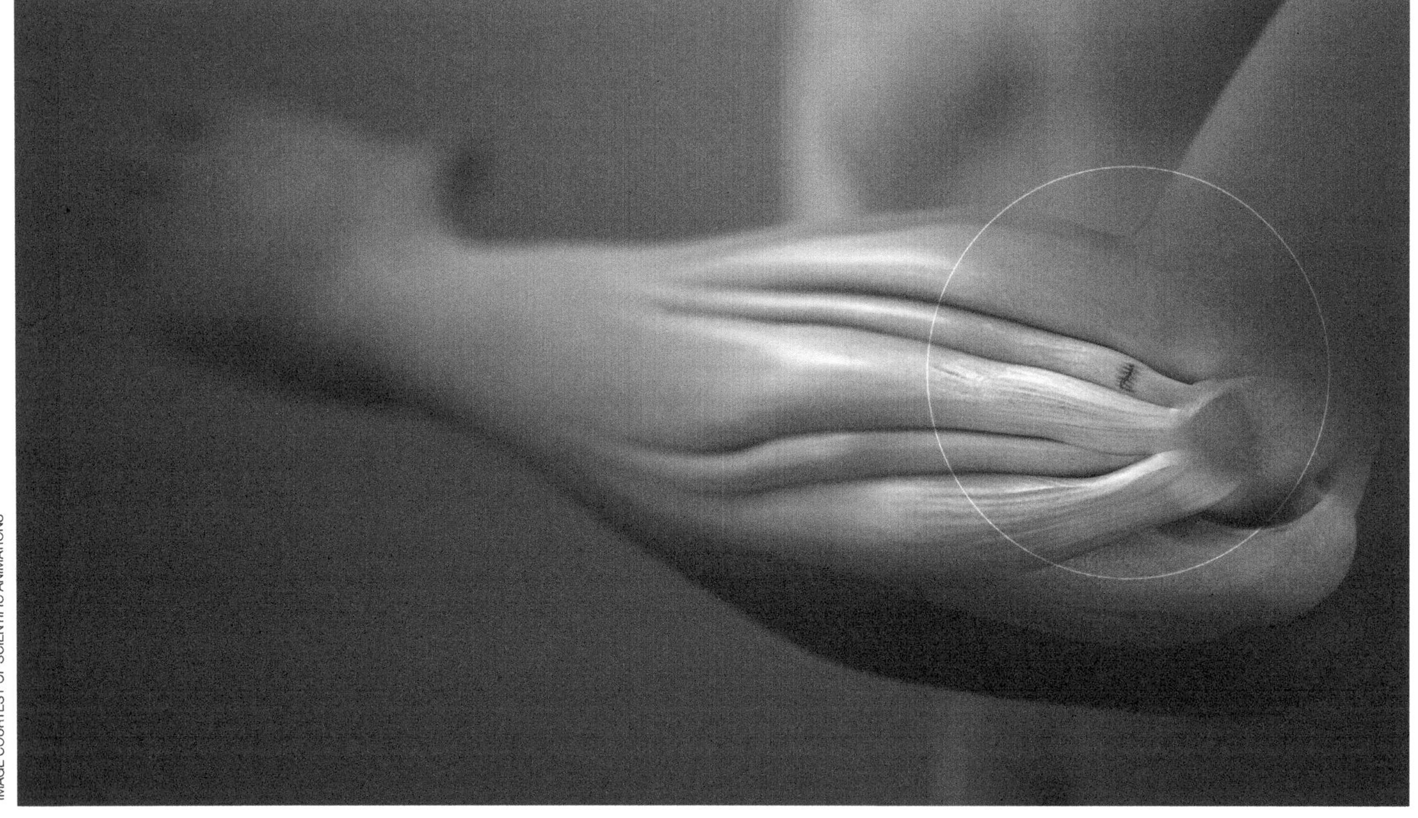

IMAGE COURTESY OF SCIENTIFIC ANIMATIONS

Tendons are like flexible ropes that connect the muscles to bones throughout the entire body. These tendons—essentially bundles of collagen fibers—are surrounded by sheaths of connective tissue, and they are extremely strong and flexible. They can endure activities with impact, such as running and jumping, but they can also be vulnerable to strain. Due to natural factors such as aging—but especially, excessive practice or overuse—tendons are susceptible to inflammation, known as tendonitis, which can cause pain and tenderness just outside of a joint. The most common causes are overuse from repetitive motion without rest, strained or unnecessary posture, and forced movements.

Related conditions may include tenosynovitis, which is tendonitis exacerbated by the inflammation of the synovial sheath covering the affected tendon. Two types of tenosynovitis, DeQuervain's tenosynovitis and trigger finger, are often caused by overuse. Trigger finger describes a condition in which a finger or thumb is locked into a bent position. DeQuervain's can also be caused by health conditions like arthritis, and it results in painful swelling in the thumb along the base by the wrist.

Carpal Tunnel

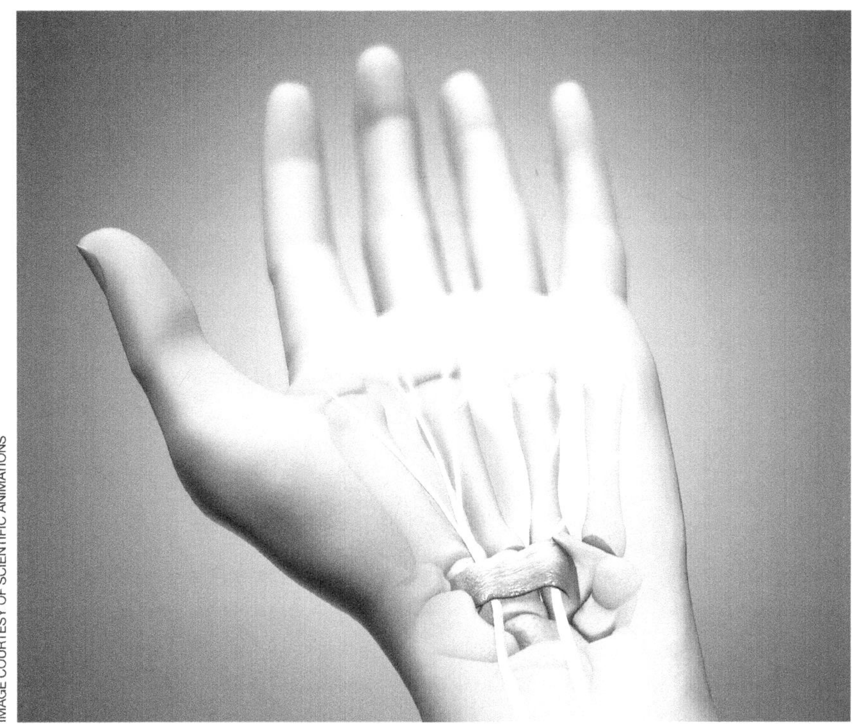

IMAGE COURTESY OF SCIENTIFIC ANIMATIONS

Carpal Tunnel Syndrome (also known as median nerve compression) is a condition caused by excessive pressure on the median nerve. This nerve is located in the arm, runs through a passage in the wrist (the carpal tunnel), and ultimately extends into the hand. The median nerve is responsible for the movement and feeling in the thumb, index, middle, and ring fingers. Excessive pressure on the nerve often results in numbness or tingling sensations, burning, itching, or general weakness (e.g., inability to grasp or hold onto an object).

As with other afflictions, carpal tunnel syndrome is typically caused by overuse and repetitive motion. People with smaller hands, wrists, and carpal tunnels may be more prone to injury, but anyone who uses excessive repetitive motion or maintains a static posture—such as playing guitar, working on a computer keyboard, or sleeping with the wrists bent—is susceptible.

Focal Dystonia

Dystonia is a disorder that can cause muscles to move or spasm involuntarily and is most often observed in musicians as focal dystonia (occurring in one specific part of the body). There are several different types of dystonia that affect various areas of the body, and while it's not exactly clear what the cause is, many doctors and researchers believe it involves problems with the brain communicating with nerve cells. Dystonia may be genetic and/or linked to other medical problems such as a brain injury or stroke.

Musician's dystonia is known as a task-specific dystonia and is commonly attributed to repetitive motion or specific activity such as playing an instrument. Symptoms aren't usually painful, but they typically show up as one or more fingers curling in (or extending out) uncontrollably while the musician is playing. In his book *Playing with Ease*, classical guitarist David Leisner documents his years-long battle with focal dystonia, ultimately curing himself and helping many other musicians recalibrate their playing by focusing on larger muscle groups and ergonomics.

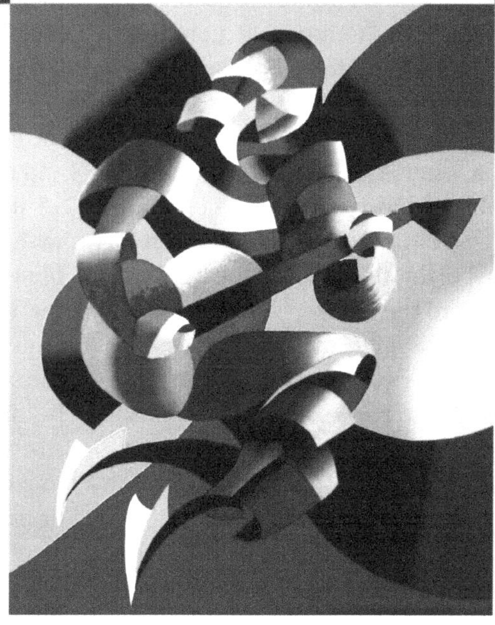

Tennis elbow, or lateral epicondylitis, is caused by repetitive motion

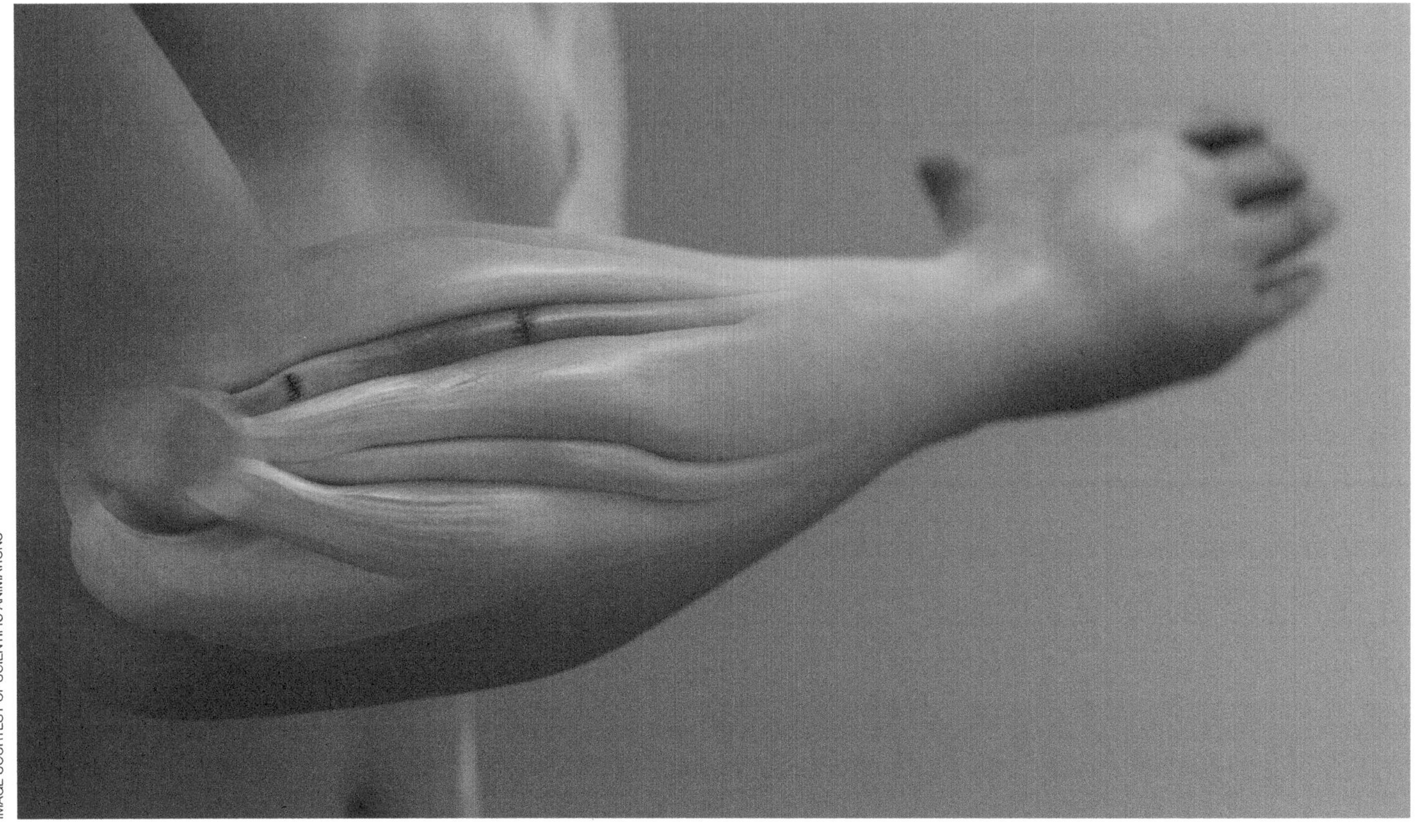

IMAGE COURTESY OF SCIENTIFIC ANIMATIONS

Arms, Shoulders, and Upper Thoracic Outlet

Another type of tendonitis is lateral epicondylitis, also known as tennis elbow, which is the most common reason for pain in the elbow area. Like other forms of tendonitis, the inflammation is caused by repetitive motion (e.g., a tennis racket swing) in one or both arms and typically manifests as pain, swelling, and/or redness on the outside of the elbow where the tendons connect to the bone.

Cubital tunnel syndrome is essentially the compression or entrapment of the ulnar nerve, which becomes inflamed in the elbow area and can result in the arm and/or specifically the pinky and ring fingers feeling sore and weak. This sensation is colloquially referred to as "hitting your funny bone," which sends an unpleasant electrical or tingling sensation down the arm into the fingers. A consistently pinched nerve in the elbow can result in numbness and discomfort, and it can affect the flexibility and dexterity of the pinky and ring fingers.

Bursae are small sacs filled with fluid that support or pad the bones, muscles, and tendons along the joints in the shoulders, elbows, knees, and throughout the body. Bursitis, the inflammation of these bursae, can cause significant pain in the affected area, especially when touched or pressed. Repetitive motion or prolonged positions can put excessive pressure on the bursae near a joint. In addition to playing the guitar, improperly carrying heavy gear or not warming up prior to strenuous activities can strain the shoulders and knees.

The thoracic outlet is the area between the bottom of the neck and upper chest/back, where bundles of nerves, muscles, and blood vessels come together and pass through to the shoulders and arms. Thoracic outlet syndrome is the compression of nerves in this area, which causes numbness and tingling in the arms and hands, and pain when the shoulders are lifted. As with other compression syndromes, repetitive stress is a common cause. But poor posture—especially slumping of the shoulders—can also be a risk factor.

Neck and Back Issues

Neck pain, which is extremely common, can be caused by something as simple as sitting or sleeping with the head in a prolonged and compromised position that stresses the neck. It can also be caused by long hours on a computer, at a workbench, reading music while playing guitar, or watching screens in uncomfortable positions. Symptoms may include stiffness, muscle aches or spasms, or even a mild headache. The neck's essential function is to support the considerable weight (10–12 pounds!) of the head on top of the spine, sometimes amusingly referred to as a bowling ball on a stick. Neck pain can also be caused by nerve compression from herniated disks or bone spurs in the vertebrae branching out into the neck.

Back pain can occur in the upper, middle, or lower back regions, and it can significantly affect one's playing. It can be experienced as chronic pain or stiffness anywhere from the neck down to the base of the spine; it can also make it difficult for one to stand up straight without muscle spasms. Spinal cord injury, which can be very serious, requires immediate medical attention. Damage to the spine may be experienced as symptoms such as numbness, tingling, or significant weakness in the groin or legs.

Herniated disks are common in the lower back just above the hips. Symptoms include sharp pain throughout the back and even down into the legs triggered by standing up quickly or bending over to pick up something, like an instrument or amp. This sharp pain is often exacerbated by bending at the waist and coughing, which causes compression on the surrounding nerves.

Nerve compression, also known as a pinched nerve, is a type of damage that occurs when excessive pressure is placed upon one or more nerves. Two common causes include repetitive motion and holding a specific area of the body in a static position for too long. Without the protection of extra soft tissue, nerves that pass through smaller spaces in the body (e.g., the carpal tunnel) are more vulnerable to inflammation caused by being pressed between tendons and bone. Nerves compression at the base of the spine often results in low back pain or neck pain that moves through the shoulders and arms. Other symptoms may include numbness, tingling, and/or a pins-and-needles burning sensation.

Sciatica refers to pain that travels from the lower back into the backs of both legs through the sciatic nerve. It can be caused by a herniated disk in the lower lumbar region of the spine. This condition is common among people who sit for long periods, such as truck drivers and office workers, and it can affect guitarists who tend to practice, teach, and even perform while sitting down.

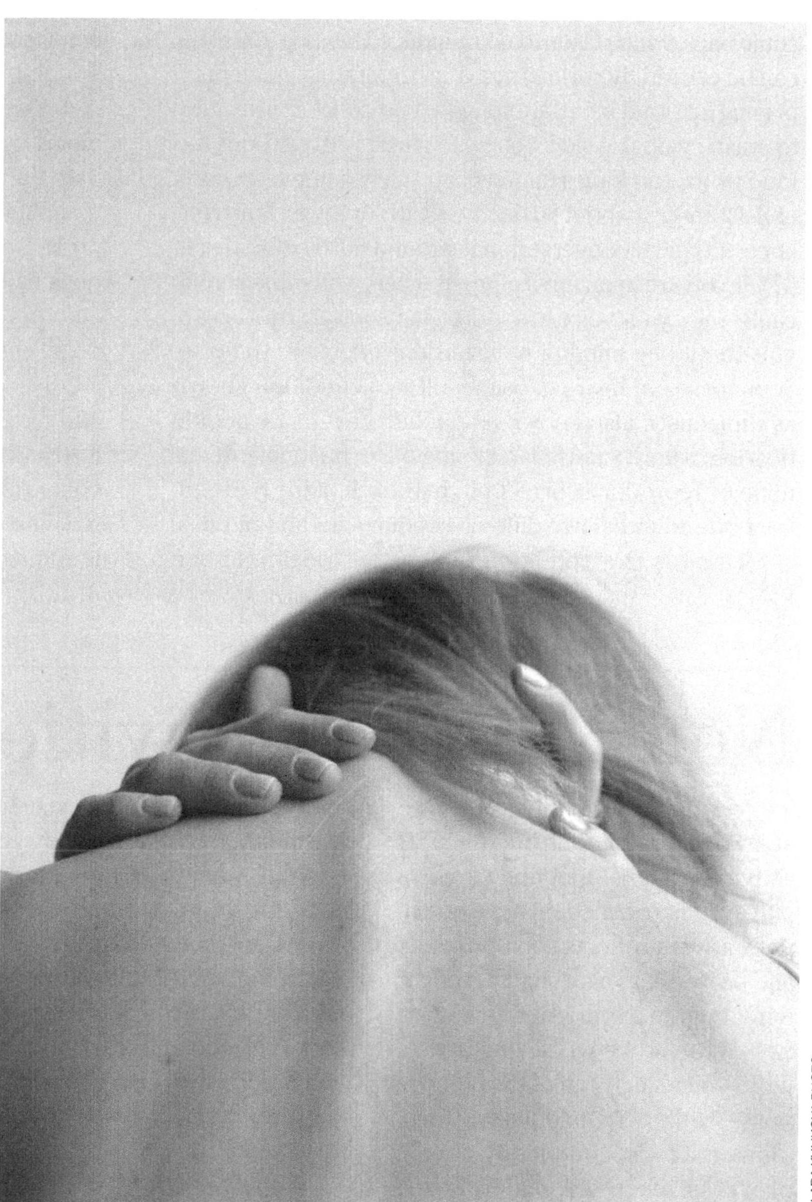

KLARA KULIKOVA PHOTO

Ear Health and Hearing Damage

The ear is comprised of three essential parts: the outer, middle, and inner ear. Each of these parts has distinct functions of transmitting and converting sound waves to signals that the brain receives. The eardrum, located between the outer and middle ear, allows sounds to vibrate and travel into the inner ear, where they pass through a spiral-shaped organ containing fluid called the cochlea. The cochlea hosts nerve cells attached to thousands of tiny little hairs called cilia, which discharge electrical impulses that travel through the auditory nerve to the brain.

When the ears are subjected to excessive loudness over time, the cilia are eventually sheared off and do not come back, which leads to noise-induced hearing loss. This can be caused by various activities: operating machinery, playing in a loud band, attending a loud concert, proximity to crash cymbals, and listening to music with ear buds too loud or for too long. Humans can safely listen to sounds consistently at about 80 decibels (dB) or lower. For reference, a typical conversation is around 50–60 dB (see pg. 37). If you are in an environment where you must significantly raise your voice to speak to someone at arm's length, you should be mindful of hazardous exposure to noise. Some cases of hearing loss result in a condition known as diplacusis, also known as pitch distortion or double hearing, where a musician or singer can no longer determine or reproduce correct pitch as each of the two ears hear one sound in two different frequencies and pitches.

Tinnitus is a condition of constant ringing in one or both ears, and while it varies in frequency and loudness—often more noticeable in quiet environments—it is a permanent condition. It is not a serious health condition but can certainly cause significant frustration and even psychological distress, especially for musicians and recording engineers. While it's possible other factors may lead to tinnitus (e.g., ear infections, sudden head trauma, temporomandibular joint and muscle disorders), far and away the most common cause of tinnitus is prolonged exposure over time to loud sounds and/or music. It is thought that once the cilia in your ears are destroyed, random electrical pulses are sent to the brain, causing inner ear noise ranging from a low, rumbling sound to a high-pitched squeal. It is also thought that lifestyle factors such as smoking, alcohol use, obesity, and high blood pressure may also contribute to and/or exacerbate tinnitus symptoms.

The next chapter will explore a variety of resources, preventative measures, solutions, and practice suggestions to avoid and/or deal with these physical, nerve, and auditory afflictions, but an overarching theme is to avoid doing any one activity, in the same way, for too long or too loudly. Your guitar should be an extension of your body, and indeed, your body and ears are extensions of your instrument. In a sense, your body, mind, and guitar should come together in a way that is ergonomic and efficient to ensure the best possible musical experience, with the least possible risk of cumulative- or noise-induced injury.

Non-Musical Activities

It is equally important to create an awareness of your non-musical activities (NMAs) that don't involve playing guitar but could have potentially adverse effects on your hands and body. Years ago, I had a student who began experiencing severe carpal tunnel in his picking hand's wrist—seemingly out of the blue. He possessed a very fluid picking technique that was completely devoid of excessive tension, and he hadn't changed his approach to playing or practicing at all. When I started asking him what else was going on in his life, he mentioned that he had recently started a new job. Being a college student, he took whatever job he could, and in this case, it was working in a butchery cutting large pieces of meat for hours at a time with no break. Needless to say, I told him to find another job! He did, and within a couple of weeks, his wrist was back to normal.

Another guitarist friend who was suffering from carpal tunnel in both hands discovered he had a habit of sleeping with both hands curled under the pillow, wrists fully flexed inward. These types of habits can be easily overlooked yet may increase the risk of injury. Another common culprit is long hours of work (e.g., writing and notating music) on a computer keyboard. Just as you should warm up and take frequent breaks while playing guitar, the same goes for any activity that involves impact and/or repetitive motion in the hands, wrists, arms, or back.

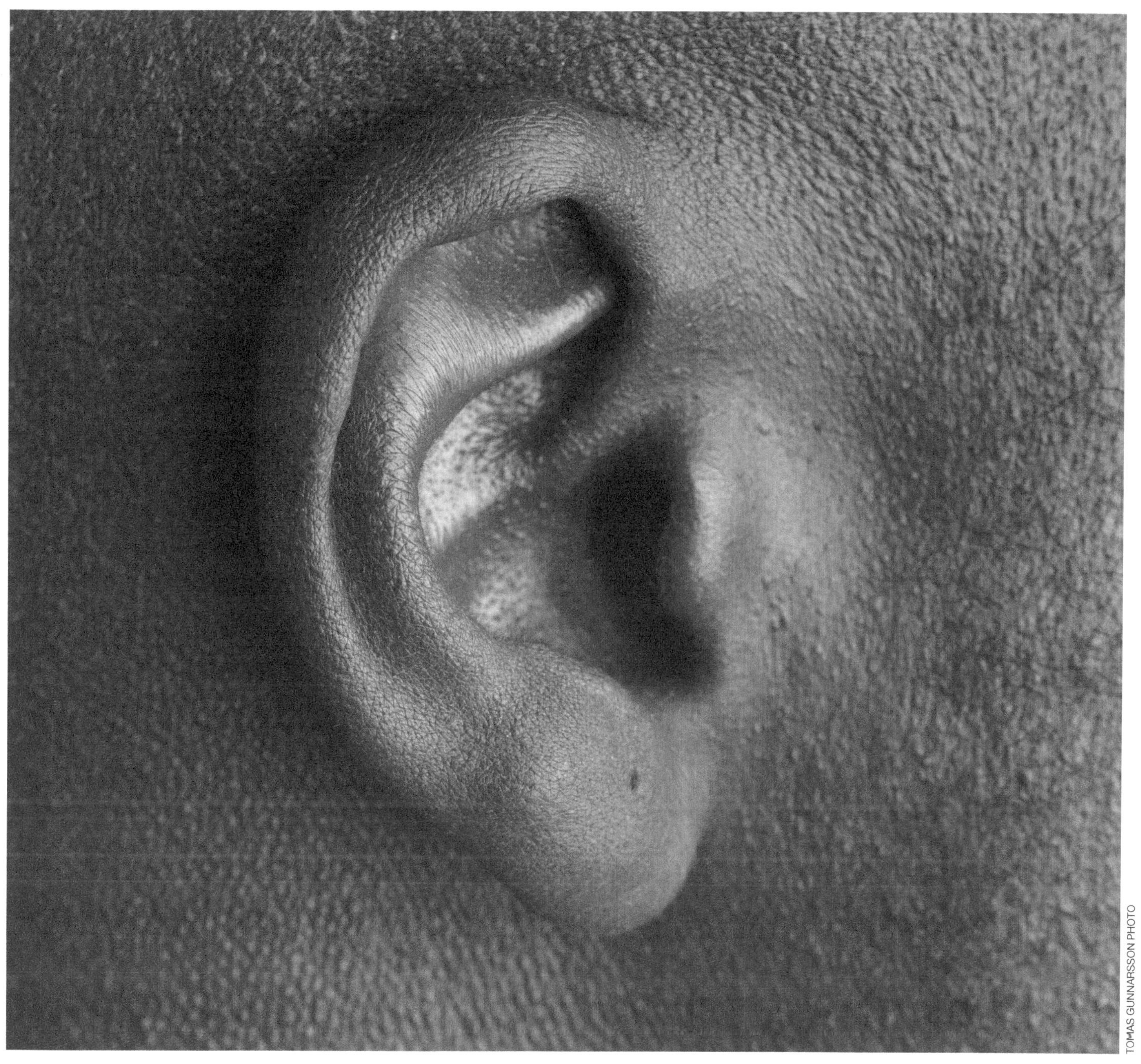

TOMAS GUNNARSSON PHOTO

Noise and Decibel Levels

According to the Centers for Disease Control and Prevention, prolonged exposure to noise above 70–80 dB can cause gradual damage that affects hearing. Here are some basic reference points in decibels.

Obviously, it's best to avoid exposure to the louder examples. But you can take precaution by wearing high-quality ear protection when operating machinery, attending a loud concert, etc. and by installing a decibel meter app on your smartphone or watch.

Whisper	30 dB
Refrigerator or air conditioner hum	40 dB
Normal conversation	50-60 dB
Lawnmowers and leaf blowers	80–95 dB
Motorcycle	95–100 dB
Live music venues and concerts	105–120 dB
Proximity to siren	120 dB
Firecrackers and gunshots	140–175 dB

CHAPTER THREE

Prevention, Solutions, and Resources for Wellness

Playing guitar indeed involves several physical demands, each of which can contribute to overuse injuries if not managed properly. Whether it's through flatpicking, strumming, playing fingerstyle, fretting, or simply holding the instrument, these activities all require repetitive motions that can strain muscles and joints. Although learning new chords, scales, melodic lines, and songs is essential for growth as a musician, overdoing it or practicing with poor technique can also increase the risk of injury.

Additionally, factors such as age, engagement in non-musical activities, and previous injuries can impact a guitarist's physical ability. As musicians get older, they may experience changes in flexibility, strength, and dexterity, which can affect their playing. Non-musical activities that involve repetitive motions or physical strain can also contribute to the risk of injury. Old injuries, whether related to playing guitar or not, can further complicate a guitarist's ability to play comfortably and safely.

The previous chapter provided an overview of the various types of idiosyncratic injuries that can affect guitarists, including hearing loss. This chapter will explore solutions, resources, and measures of prevention to help guitarists avoid or manage these injuries, ensuring they can continue to play music comfortably and healthily.

Prelude No. 3

A13
E♭9
D9
A♭13
A13
B♭13
Em11
E♭9
let ring throughout
D9
G13
C♯7♯9
F♯7♯5
C9
B7♯9
E13
E7♯9
A7
C7
B7
F7
E7
A7
D7
A7
G13
E9
A9

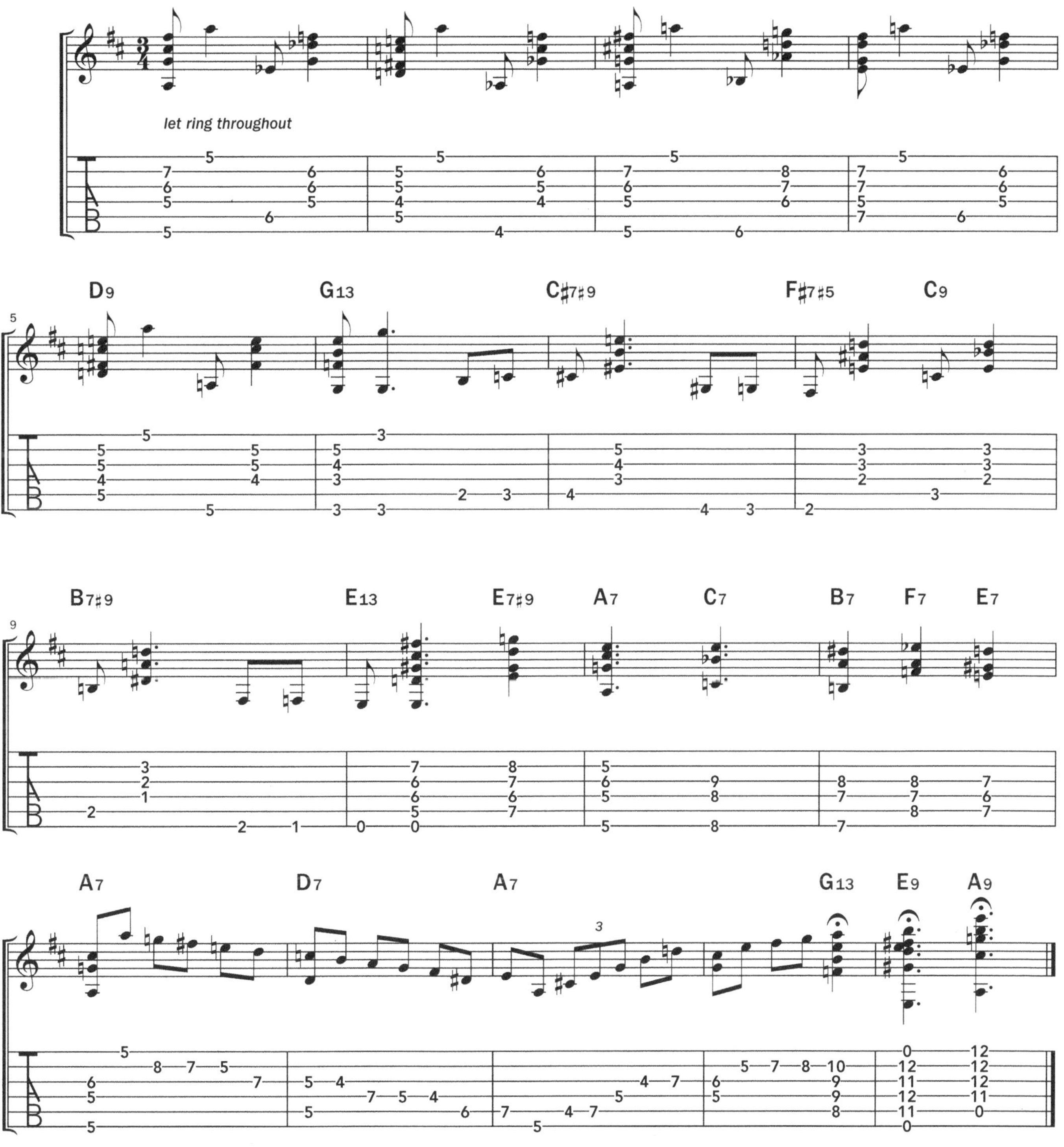

Prevention

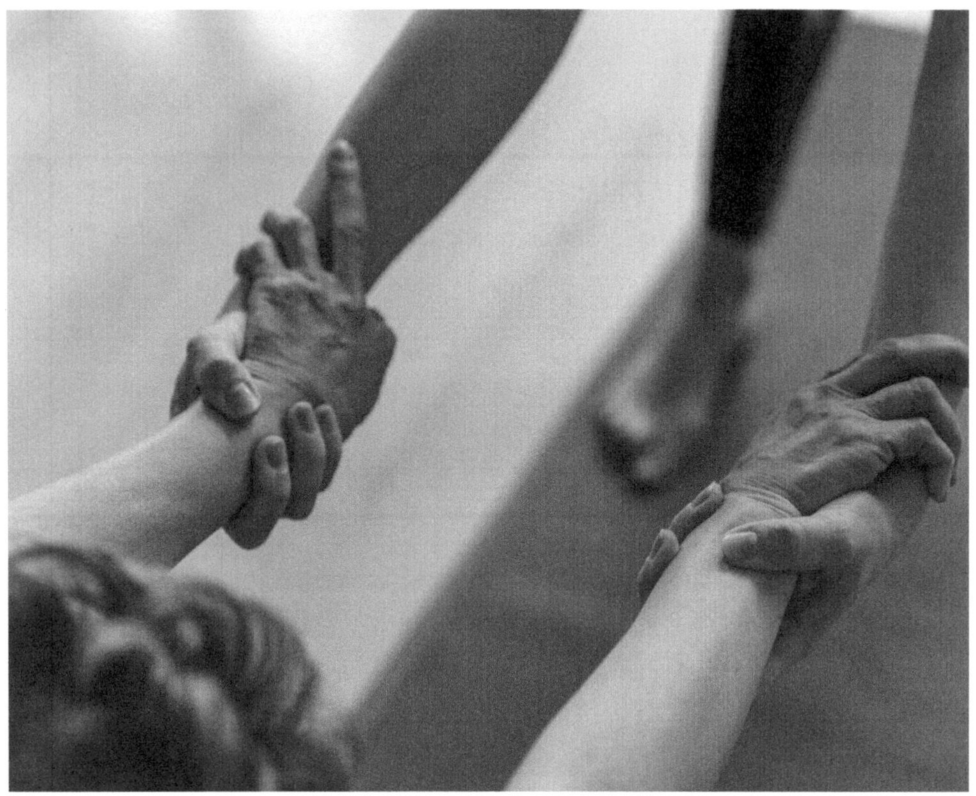
RASPOPOVA MARINA PHOTO

It's crucial to prioritize injury prevention from the outset of your guitar journey, as the first injury can set back progress significantly. Prevention begins with cultivating a deep self-awareness during your practice sessions. This includes paying attention to your posture, ensuring you use proper technique without strain, monitoring the frequency and duration of your practice sessions, and applying ergonomic principles.

Maintaining good general health is a recurring theme, and it doesn't require extreme measures like daily gym workouts. Simple habits like stretching throughout the day, especially before and after practice, can greatly reduce the risk of injury. The stretches detailed in Chapter 1 are akin to those recommended by physical or occupational therapists for rehabilitation after injury, making them highly effective preventive measures.

It is essential to incorporate warm-up routines both with and without your guitar before each practice session. Even if time is limited, these routines prepare your muscles and joints for the demands of playing. Similarly, a cool-down period at the end of your session, which could involve reviewing materials, improvising over different rhythms, or playing familiar songs for enjoyment, helps to gradually ease tension in your hands and body. Gentle stretches for your fingers, hands, and arms afterward further aid in relaxation and recovery.

Developing self-awareness while playing is another vital aspect of prevention. Recording yourself and watching for signs of tension in your back, neck, shoulders, or arms can provide valuable feedback. Any discomfort or fatigue noticed after playing indicates areas where adjustments may be necessary.

Visualizing different parts of your body during play can also help identify areas of tension or poor posture. This mindfulness allows you to adjust your technique and posture to achieve effortless playing. The goal is to cultivate a playing style that supports musical intensity without unnecessary strain, promoting longevity and enjoyment in your guitar practice.

Treatments and Options for Therapy

Throughout this book, you will notice common and recurring themes regarding the avoidance and treatment of most repetitive strain and cumulative trauma injuries. These include taking frequent breaks, periods of rest (if injured), practicing with consistency, applying ergonomics, creating an awareness of the body and posture, recognizing excessive tension, a solid stretching and warm-up routine, and maintaining strength and flexibility through low-impact exercises. Here are some additional guidelines for treating cumulative trauma disorders, which in most cases are not serious but simply require rest, relaxation, and perhaps a reassessment and recalibration of your physical approach to the instrument. Remember always to consult a medical expert and/or your primary care physician in the event of any signs of injury, discomfort, or pain.

Tendonitis

The first thing to do is rest and discontinue the activities that are causing inflammation as soon and as much as possible. Inflammation is typically caused by overuse, so in addition to cutting back and/or ceasing activities, you can treat symptoms with ice packs and/or heat, along with an anti-inflammatory medicine such as Ibuprofen. Some musicians have tried steroid injections, with mixed results, but it's not an ideal method of treatment. For chronic tendon irritation, platelet-rich plasma (PRP) treatments have been shown to help. If symptoms persist, it's advisable to discuss other options with your primary care doctor.

Ideally, symptoms will dissipate after a brief period of rest (e.g., a few days to a week, depending on the severity), stretching, and/or physical therapy if necessary, followed by a thorough assessment of what caused the initial inflammation. Long-term inflammation, however, may lead to a torn tendon, which typically requires surgery.

Carpal Tunnel Syndrome

Like tendonitis, carpal tunnel can also occur from gripping things like a phone or guitar neck too tightly. Symptoms often include tenderness and pain when bending the wrist and/or tapping on the nerves that pass through the wrist. Cold or ice packs can help reduce swelling. Another common treatment is using a splint at night while sleeping, which keeps the wrist in a straight position and can help alleviate symptoms of numbness and tingling in the nerve. If symptoms persist, see a medical professional who will perform a physical exam or ultrasound to assess the tendons and nerves.

Thoracic Outlet Syndrome

This syndrome, which results from nerve compression between the neck and arms, can cause pain in the neck and shoulders, extreme weakness in the arms, and numbness in the fingers. Diagnosis of thoracic outlet syndrome is often confirmed by an MRI, ultrasound, or CT scan. If diagnosed early, treatment can be relatively simple, involving physical therapy and medications such as muscle relaxants and/or anti-inflammatory medicines. If a blood clot is detected, however, your doctor may prescribe anticoagulant medicines.

Sciatica and Back Pain

Dealing with sciatica symptoms at home should involve stretching exercises (slow and smooth), along with cold packs. After a few days, you can try short intervals with a heating pad. Alternative therapies that may help include acupuncture and massage therapy—especially Trager work if the back is too sensitive to touch.

Low back pain can often be mitigated by anti-inflammatory pain relievers used in moderation, as well as topical ointments and patches that provide relief through the skin. If your pain persists, you may benefit from seeing an acupuncturist or chiropractic doctor. Physical therapy typically involves stretching and strengthening exercises, as well as an assessment of musical and non-musical activities that may be causing back pain. For guitarists, low back pain is often caused by sitting too long and/or in a compromised position (e.g., practicing, performing sitting down, driving for hours in a car)—essentially, engaging in any activity in one static position for too long without breaks or variation.

Wellness Resources and Options for Guitarists

There is an abundance of resources available to guitarists, aimed at promoting optimal health, wellness, and specific injury prevention strategies. Information about these activities and methodologies (see pg. 43) can be found online, including directories to locate local and regional certified practitioners. Here are some practices popular among professional instrumentalists and vocalists that can benefit guitarists in particular.

Alexander Technique

Developed by Australian actor F. M. Alexander in the late 19th century, the Alexander Technique is an approach that facilitates ease of movement, paying close attention to postural alignment, balance, principles of motion, interaction with everyday objects, and addressing physical complications and pains that have developed over many years due to poor habits. Through a series of group and individual lessons, students learn to recalibrate both physical and mental habits to interact with the world more efficiently, elegantly, and mindfully. Many orchestral string musicians, as well as acoustic/classical guitarists, have benefited from Alexander Technique lessons, often attributing a greater projection of sound and a more beautiful tone to newfound levels of self-awareness. The Alexander Technique is commonly offered within the curriculum of music and theatre conservatories around the world.

Feldenkrais

Moshé Feldenkrais was an engineer, athlete, and expert in ju-jitsu. After suffering a series of debilitating knee injuries with a poor prognosis for surgical success, he, like F. M. Alexander, embarked on an intensive journey of self-rehabilitation and awareness. His goal was to heal his body, leading to the development of the foundational concepts of the Feldenkrais Method. The method is taught through group lessons known as Awareness Through Movement and individual lessons called Functional Integration. In these settings, students learn principles of somatic education, biomechanics, and fluidity of movement, which can be highly beneficial for guitarists in practical terms.

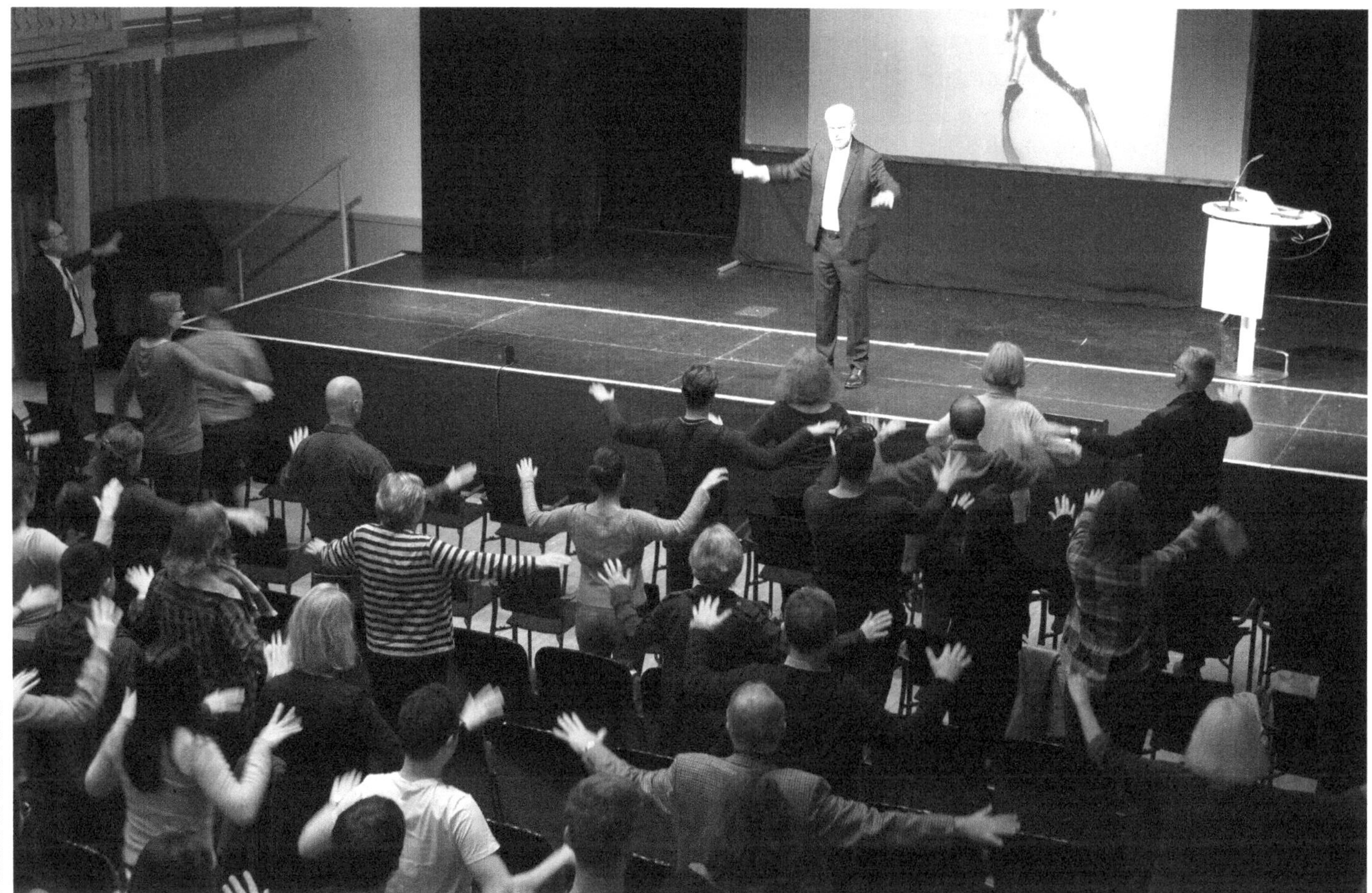

THORSTEN KRIENKE PHOTO

Lecture Demonstration: "An Introduction to the Alexander-Technique for Musicians" by Prof. Robert Britton San Francisco, 2019

Yoga

Many musicians study various forms of yoga and find their practice to be indispensable for long-term health and success playing an instrument. One caveat: Beware of extreme fad styles of yoga that impose excessive wear and tear on the wrists and other joints. Instead, opt for gentler styles and postures that do not stress parts of the body directly involved in playing guitar. There are yoga studios specifically catering to musicians and performing artists, which may be beneficial to include in your wellness routine.

Tai Chi and Qigong

Also popular among musicians worldwide is the practice of tai chi and/or qigong. Tai chi is an ancient Chinese exercise that integrates the mind and body through a series of postures and graceful movements. Health benefits may include relief of arthritis symptoms, increased flexibility, and improved balance. Some of the mental benefits are comparable to meditation, helping to cultivate a more relaxed and focused mind.

Chi, or qi, describes vital life force energy. Another popular ancient Chinese practice is qigong, which shares many similarities with tai chi. Qigong emphasizes breath work and stillness while practicing different postures, aiming to develop and circulate energy. While tai chi involves a longer series of memorized forms, some find qigong more accessible due to its simpler practice routines.

Both tai chi and qigong are excellent for people of all ages and health profiles, offering numerous benefits for guitarists such as improved balance, coordination, muscle and tendon flexibility, and enhanced joint function.

Massage Therapy and Trager Approach

Just as it does for athletes, massage therapy can yield positive results for guitarists who may be struggling with various levels and types of muscle or back pain, or simply as a supplement to a physical exercise regimen. Deep tissue, Swedish, and/or sports massage can help alleviate excessive tension and promote relaxation and blood oxygen flow, which can be especially effective for touring musicians.

The Trager Approach was developed by Milton Trager, a physician who dedicated his life to the study of physical rehabilitation and mind-body integration. A session with a certified Trager practitioner can be helpful for musicians who have acute pain in the lower back or sciatica, where traditional massage therapy may be too painful. In contrast to the direct touch and work of a massage, Trager incorporates gentle movements by holding and supporting the legs and arms slightly elevated while lying on a table, gently rotating to promote more of an internal massage. Guitarists who suffer from back pain have experienced positive results from Trager sessions.

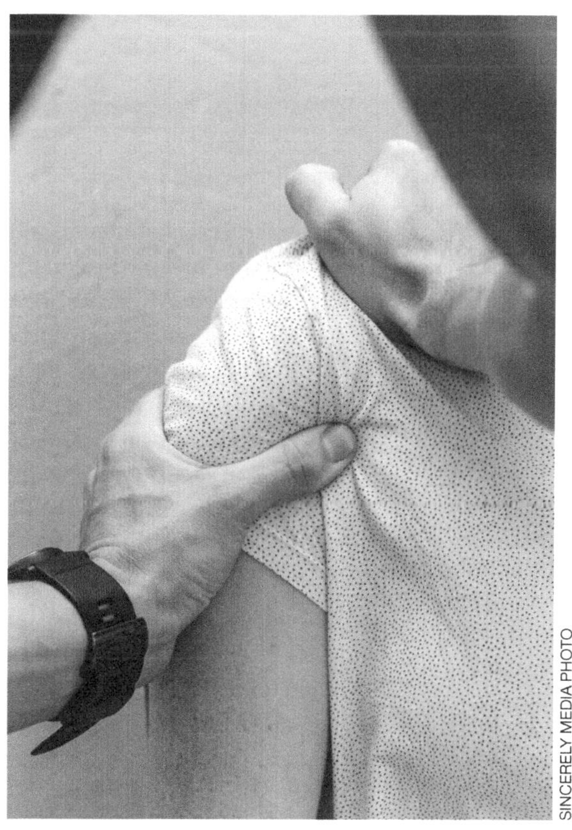

SINCERELY MEDIA PHOTO

Wellness Directory

Following is a list of online resources, many of which feature directories by state and region, to find a certified/licensed practitioner and/or classes:

The Complete Guide to the Alexander Technique
alexandertechnique.com

The Feldenkrais Method/Awareness Through Movement
feldenkrais.com

The Trager Approach
trager.com

Tai Chi
taichiforhealthinstitute.org

National Qigong Association
nqa.org/what-is-qigong

Yoga Information
nccih.nih.gov/health/yoga-what-you-need-to-know

Yoga for Musicians
yogawithadriene.com/yoga-for-musicians

Pilates
pilates.com/what-is-pilates-and-benefits

Performing Arts Medicine Association
artsmed.org

Hand Therapy for Musicians
musichandstherapy.com

Acupuncture
hopkinsmedicine.org/health/wellness-and-prevention/acupuncture

Pillars of Health

The three commonly known pillars of good health are exercise, sleep, and nutrition, all of which can seem contradictory to the lifestyle of a professional musician, touring musicians in particular. The inherent lifestyle of musicians—late-night gigs, long hours of travel, inconsistent quality of food on the road, eating late at night, and not getting enough sleep—can wreak havoc on their health. Fulfilling each of these three areas requires discipline and planning.

Exercise

Exercise options for every guitarist—whether touring artists or local working musicians—include low-impact activities such as walking, strength training, stretching, yoga, swimming, or biking. Some guitarists prefer a daily run, especially when on tour. Just 20 to 30 minutes of daily exercise can greatly improve sleep, mental clarity, confidence, and building performance endurance.

Strength training that focuses on more reps with low to medium weights can work wonders for building core muscles needed for long concerts onstage, traveling between shows, and optimizing overall performance and health. Walking is an excellent option that can be done anywhere and anytime; it's also a great way to clear the mind, visualize, and memorize songs or fretboard exercises.

Generally speaking, guitarists should engage in low-impact exercises and choose activities that do not strain the hands, wrists, fingers, neck, or any other crucial part of the body involved in playing.

Sleep

Make a commitment to getting enough sleep, especially on the road. After a show, of course, musicians are inclined to hang out, which is natural, but it's important to remember that over time, consistent lack of sleep can negatively impact performance quality. As professionals, we are obligated to give our best to each performance, and during a tour, it's crucial to prioritize good sleep whenever possible.

Nutrition

Plan to eat well on tour or when traveling to a gig. It's much easier—and more affordable—to prepare and pack your own food in advance, just as you would any other piece of gear. Some touring musicians have even retrofitted their vehicles to include equipment for food prep and cooking. When you're on the road, avoid fast-food joints or highly processed items at convenience stores; instead, stop at grocery stores that offer fresh produce and nutritious food options.

A good supply of nuts, dried and fresh fruits, leafy greens, vegetables, healthy protein snacks, whole grains, and water can go a long way in supporting and sustaining your energy levels while traveling. Choosing healthy whole foods in general will contribute to your overall well-being and performance readiness during tours.

A Classical Guitarist's Journey Through Back Pain

Jeff LaQuatra, an accomplished classical guitarist and educator who directs the guitar program at Colorado State University, experienced extreme lower back pain due to years of constant sitting during practice, performances, and teaching without proper preventative measures. This condition even prevented him from sitting down with a guitar at times. Now, he emphasizes to his students and incorporates into his own practice routine the importance of exercise, postural awareness, taking frequent breaks, and implementing alternative practice measures.

As young musicians, we often focus intensely on developing our technique and musicianship, primarily centered around our hands and fingers. However, it's crucial to recognize that practicing and performing engage the entire body, particularly placing significant stress on the lower lumbar region whether sitting or standing. There's a humorous yet poignant reference among guitarists to L-5 surgery, which refers both to the L4/L5 lumbar vertebrae and Gibson's L-5 archtop. Having undergone this serious surgery myself, I can attest that it's often avoidable.

In addition to hours spent practicing scales and arpeggios, it's essential to incorporate physical activities that suit your body's needs, focusing on strength, flexibility, and balance. Options like strength training, yoga, Pilates, and walking can be beneficial. Following a herniated disc in my L4/L5 vertebrae, I eventually opted for surgery as a last resort, which fortunately, was successful. Since then, prioritizing physical therapy, core strength training, and daily walks has helped me maintain a healthy lifestyle and approach to playing the guitar. I now practice and perform without discomfort or pain. Always remember, your body keeps score!

— *Jeff LaQuatra*

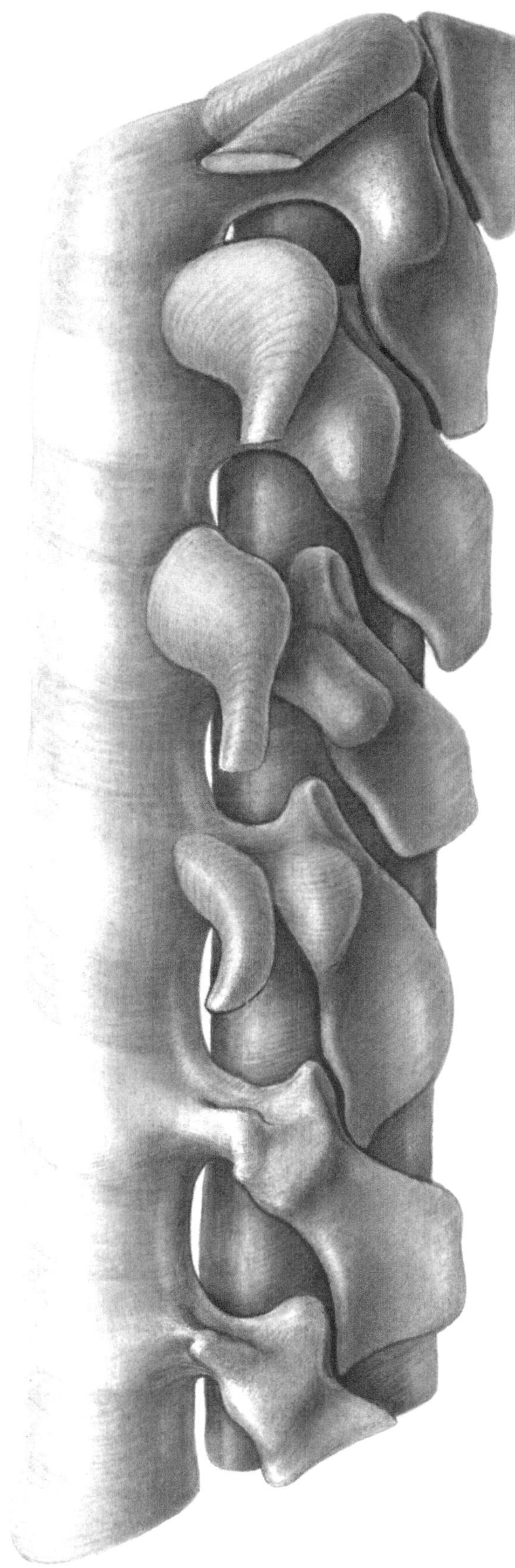

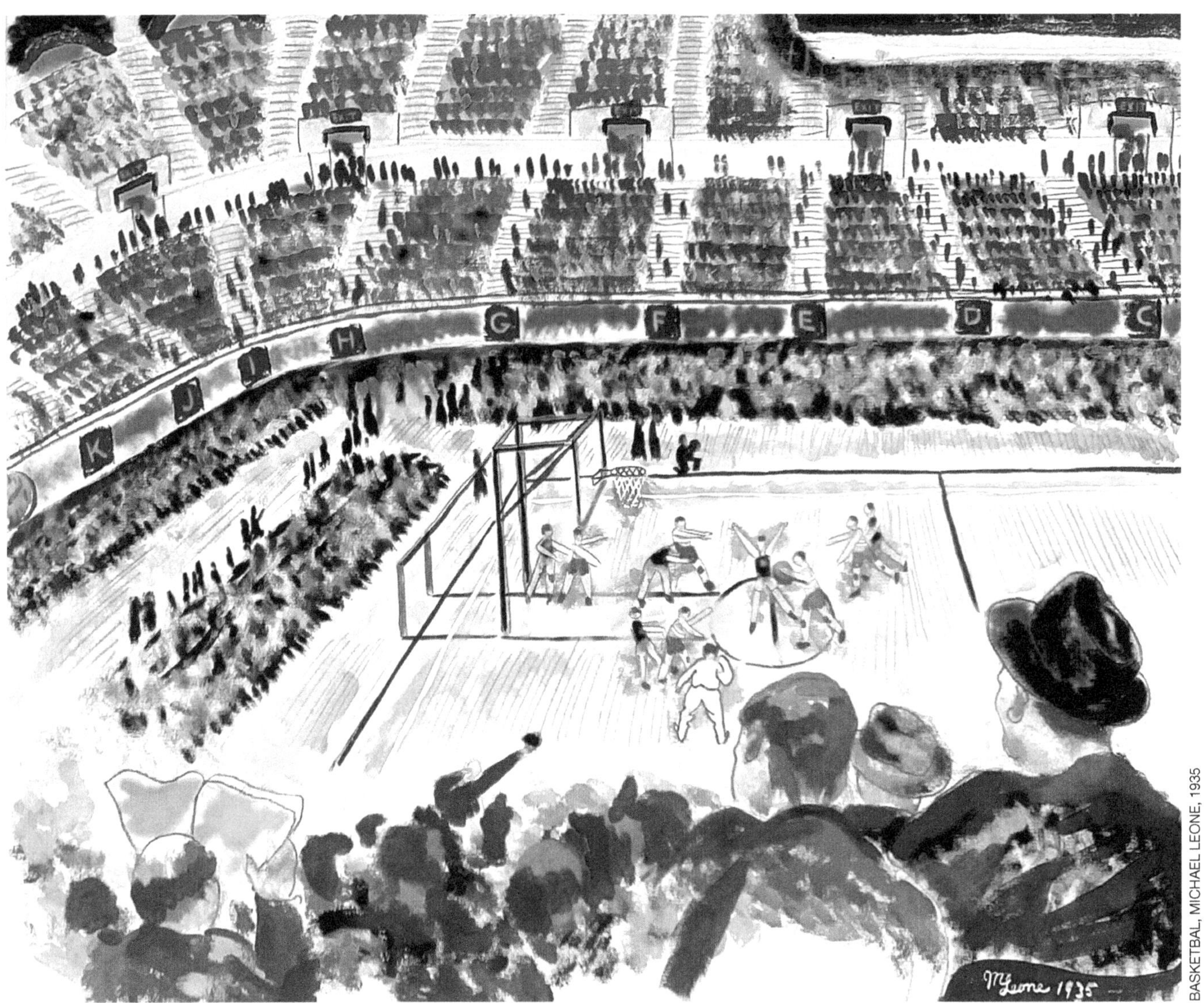

BASKETBAL, MICHAEL LEONE, 1935

The Artist as Athlete

In a way, high-level instrumentalists are like Olympic athletes on a miniaturized scale: We begin with some talent, add a large dose of determination, learn proper technique, and repeat, repeat, repeat until our muscles and neural pathways are properly developed. We train our minds, and we strive to have fun throughout the process.

Here's a tip I teach my students and always use myself: Squeeze the strings with the fretting hand only as tightly as necessary to produce a proper sound, then release the strings simply by relaxing. Many people tend to squeeze too hard and move too far. When guitarists relax the fretting hand, the tension of the strings naturally pushes the fingertips off the fretboard, muting the open strings upon release. This is a quiet and effortless way to change positions without creating distracting pull-off sounds from open strings.

If this concept is new to you, try practicing it slowly at first, initially without removing your fingertips from the strings: Squeeze, relax, squeeze, relax. As the ancient inventor Archimedes once said, "The shortest distance between two points is a straight line." Aim for your fingertips to travel as short a distance as possible between positions—avoid making triangular movements with your fingertips. Here's my suggestion: When changing chords, relax the previous position first, muting the strings as you release. Then, visualize the new chord, and with enough repetition, your fingertips will move nearly effortlessly in a mostly straight line directly to the new position on the fretboard.

This approach is efficient and smooth, enhancing both the sound of your music and your ability to play comfortably for extended periods. Combined with proper eating, sleeping, and exercise habits, it has allowed me to play successfully and without pain for many hours a day over several decades.

—Mark Hanson

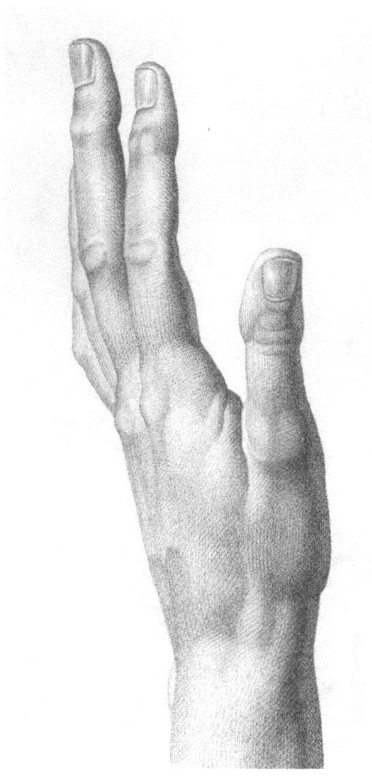

PRP Treatments

After 50 years of playing guitar, I suddenly began experiencing hand pain. An ultrasound revealed torn cartilage, ligaments, and tendons in both wrists. Despite trying chiropractic, massage, and acupuncture, which didn't provide relief, I sought treatment at a sports medicine clinic offering PRP (platelet-rich plasma) therapy. This involves centrifuging the patient's blood to concentrate platelets in plasma, which is then injected into damaged tissues.

However, the initial PRP treatment didn't fully heal my injuries, possibly due to my age (65 at the time). My doctor recommended a second PRP treatment, this time incorporating some of my fat tissue. This thickened the plasma, helping it stay localized rather than draining away. Importantly, fat tissue contains stem cells, which may have contributed to my complete healing two months later, after over a year of being unable to play guitar.

—Mike Doolin

Sound Advice

Kyle Knuppel is a board-certified physician who also holds degrees in voice, guitar, and composition. Here's some of his advice on the prevention and management of cumulative trauma syndromes that tend to affect guitarists:

Cumulative Trauma Disorder (CTD) involves what many would presume: pain, swelling, numbness, and tingling, which are all common presenting symptoms of musculoskeletal injury. Many of my colleagues in physical therapy, occupational therapy, orthopedics, audiology, otolaryngology, and integrative medicine recommend patients be seen sooner rather than later. Delays in care may complicate recovery.

Something as simple as a telehealth appointment can happen in a matter of minutes, allowing for a care plan that may include standard investigations and treatments, with potential referrals to specialists if needed. This approach is equally important for our psychological well-being. Emotional and physical healing begins when we acknowledge that we're struggling. Being patient and gentle with oneself while exploring the causes and treatments for injury is paramount.

Acknowledging the pain or disabling signs and symptoms is crucial. Listen to your body as attentively as you do your guitar playing. Just as you identify strengths and areas for improvement in your music, take time to pinpoint where you notice the physical problem. It's not always where we initially expect. In medicine, when evaluating musculoskeletal pain, we often say, "Inspect the joint above and the joint below." For instance, in the hand, which consists of 27 bones and corresponding joints from the wrist to the fingers, there can be indirect origins of disorder that are not immediately apparent. Even the smallest deviations from normal can lead to disability.

Hand and wrist pain can stem from both neurological and musculoskeletal issues. Initially, see a primary care clinician for a physical exam and assessment. This may involve bloodwork to rule out underlying inflammatory, hormonal, electrolyte imbalances, or nutrient deficiencies, among other factors. Additionally, imaging such as X-rays, ultrasound, CT, or MRI scans may be performed to help diagnose the condition definitively.

Depending on the findings, a guitarist experiencing musculoskeletal or neurological complaints may be referred to specialists in physical or occupational medicine, sports medicine, neurology, or hand surgery. Osteopaths, integrative medicine practitioners, acupuncturists, chiropractors, and others offer various forms of treatment that often complement standard allopathic care plans. Choosing clinicians experienced in integrative medicine—and particularly those who work with musicians—can help navigate this often-overwhelming process safely.

The bottom line: If it hurts, rest. And when you think you've rested enough, rest some more. Rest does not mean immobilization. We rarely immediately immobilize people with overuse injuries. Complete immobilization can lead to muscle atrophy and increase the risk of further injury. Given the diverse conditions contributing to CTD, in addition to rest, consider first-line therapies such as ice or heat, based on the advice of your physician. Over-the-counter medications like Ibuprofen or Naproxen Sodium (NSAIDs) can provide relief for minor aches and pains throughout the day by reducing inflammation. Acetaminophen (Tylenol), while not an anti-inflammatory, can alleviate discomfort for many. If you experience a precipitating event such as direct injury, worsening pain, or unfamiliar sensations, seeking expert advice promptly is advisable.

Physical injury often takes an emotional toll, especially among artists. During periods of rest and recovery, explore other avenues of creativity such as composition, production, and listening. In times of physical adversity, we can find strength in other aspects of our artistry.

—Kyle Knuppel, M.D.

CHAPTER FOUR

Mental Wellness and Growth Mindset

"We suffer more in imagination than in reality."
–LUCIUS SENECA

The mind can be an incredible asset—or obstacle—to practice, performance, and musical and/or technical improvement. Our experience depends on how we cultivate our mindsets to embrace optimism, patience, growth, and acceptance. Just like learning new music, working on mindset takes practice—plus some good perspective and inspiration that can help lift you up in challenging times.

This chapter will explore different ways to promote a healthy and positive mindset, which go a long way toward helping your musical success. We'll explore strategies to deal with performance anxiety, unhealthy competition, and the inner critic.

We'll also look at ways to use visualization techniques that strengthen concentration, memorization, and musical focus. Keeping a practice journal can keep the mind centered, cognizant of growth, and will help to develop patience with yourself and your playing, empowering you to resist the temptation of allowing pervasive negativity into your practice and performances.

Prelude No. 4

Dm Gm Am Dm C F
5
B♭maj7 E7♭9 A7♭9
9
B7♭9 E7♭9 A7♭9 Dm
13
D7♭9 Gm E7♭9 A7♭9 D

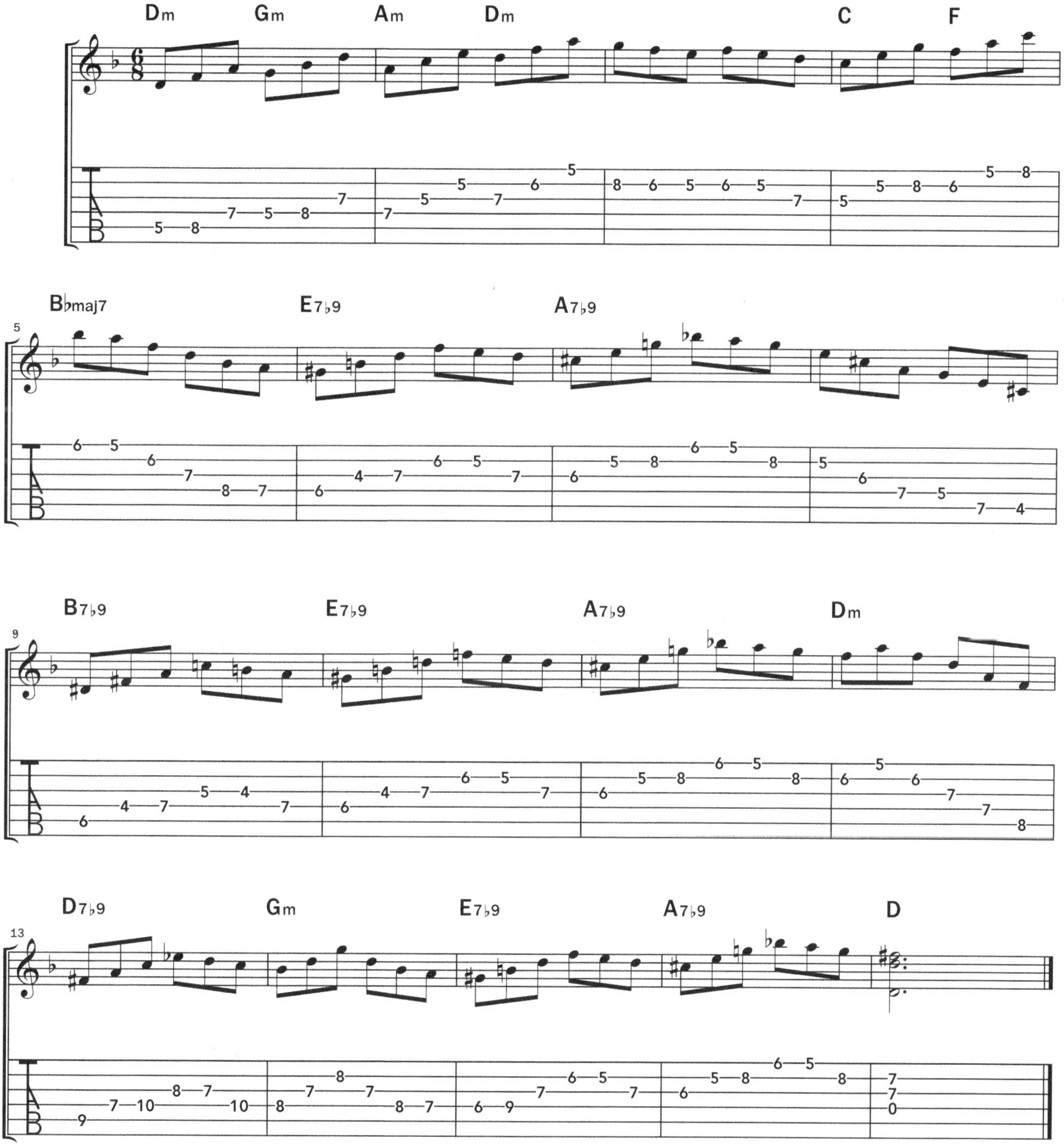

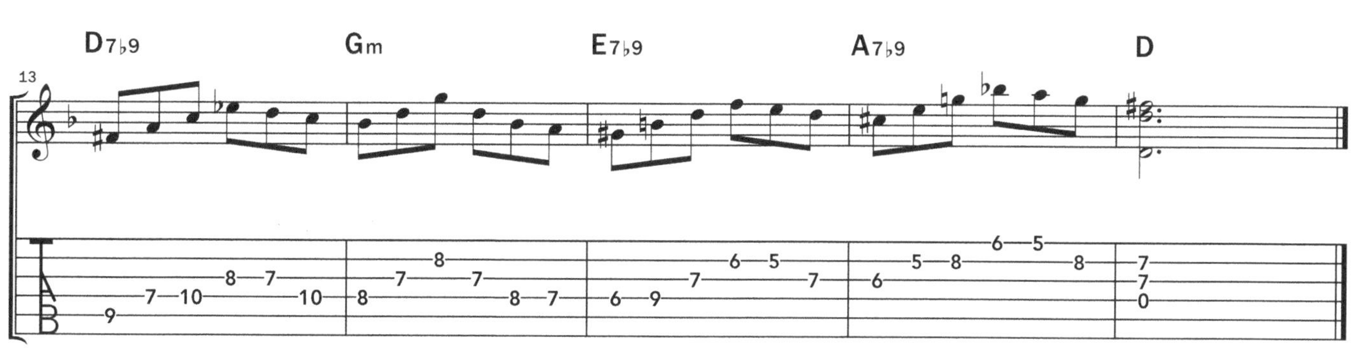

Establishing a Healthy Mindset

Music is art, not a competition. Although we may all recognize the truth and value in that statement, it can be challenging at times to stay positive when it feels like everyone is making progress except you. And let's face it—playing the guitar isn't easy at first! Indeed, legendary jazz guitarist Wes Montgomery once noted, "The guitar is such a hard instrument... because it takes years to start working with it, and it looks like everybody else is moving on the instrument but you. Then when you find a cat that's really playing, you'll always find that he's been playing a long time, you can't get around it."

It takes perseverance—and sometimes stubbornness—to break through ruts, even though it doesn't seem like it'll ever pay off. As Montgomery says, "When you find guitar players that are playing, you'll find out that at one time they never cared if they never played, they were going to keep on until they did. After a period of time the beginning player will hear a little difference in his playing, and that little inspiration is enough to go further, and the first thing you know, you won't back out. The biggest problem is getting started. Then later every time you hear guitar players everybody plays more than you. And those things are not very inspirational, they're pretty discomforting. And then somebody says, 'Why don't you put that thing down, you're not doing anything with it.' Well, that's no help. And you'll find more people against you than for you, until you get started. Then you'll find more with you than against you."

Jazz guitar great Jim Hall was once asked if he was self-critical, to which he answered, "I am, but I do feel good about my playing. The instrument keeps me humble. Sometimes I pick it up and it seems to say, 'No, you can't play today.' I keep at it anyway, though."

Keep in mind that these are honest comments from two of the greatest guitarists in American musical history. Everyone struggles at some point, but the most important thing is to keep striving and to distance yourself from potentially damaging external or internal criticism. The goal is to cultivate a healthy perspective regarding our playing and progress compared to others, balancing ambition and passion with patience, confidence with humility, and perseverance with letting go. Part of establishing a growth mindset is recognizing the long haul. You can easily spend a lifetime engaged with music and still have room for improvement. This is a beautiful practice that is spiritual in nature; in fact, the word "practice" is both a verb and a noun. A practice is a habit, a custom, and an ongoing work in progress. Life is a journey—practice is the destination. It's a constant state of movement and flow.

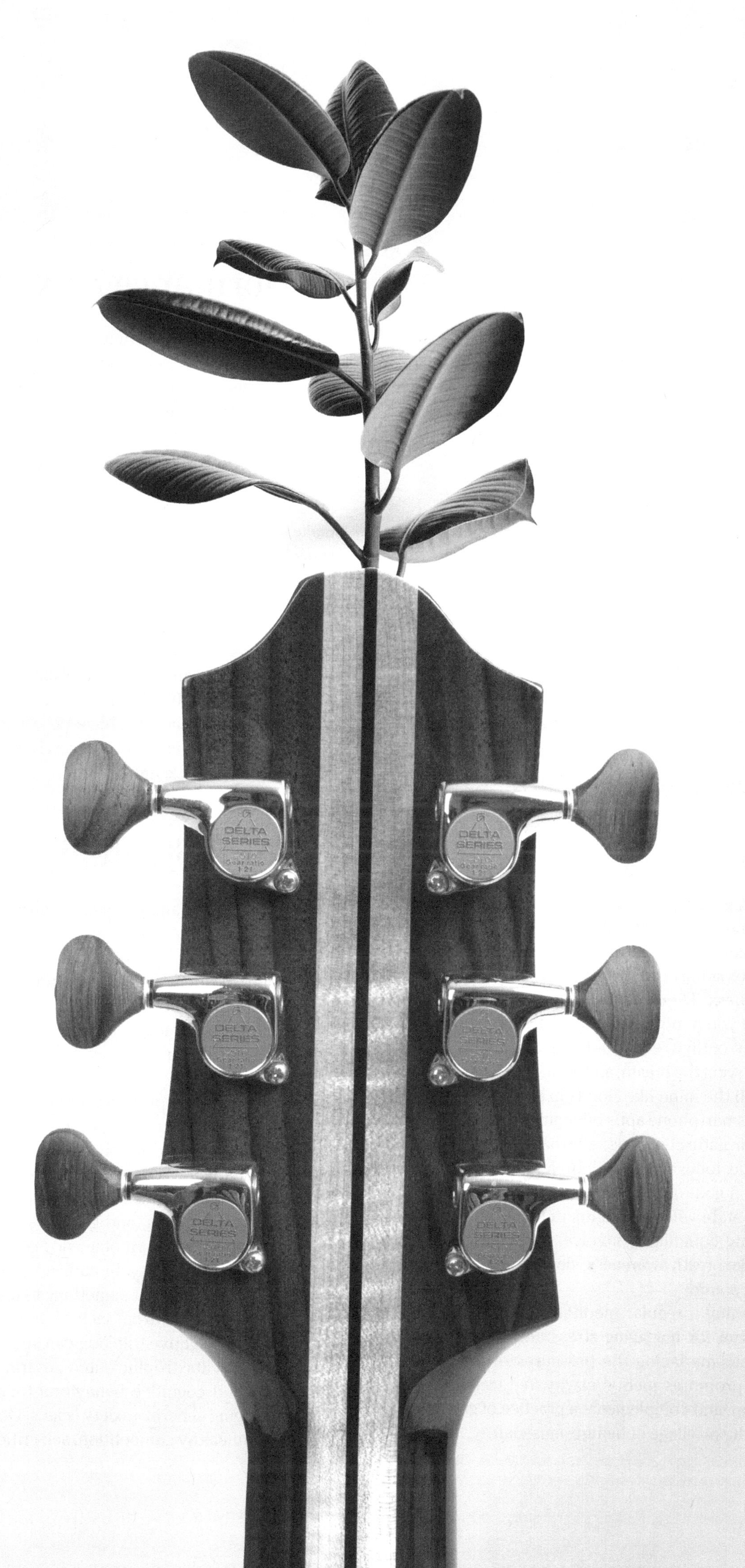
DELTA SERIES
DELTA SERIES
DELTA SERIES
DELTA SERIES
DELTA SERIES
DELTA SERIES

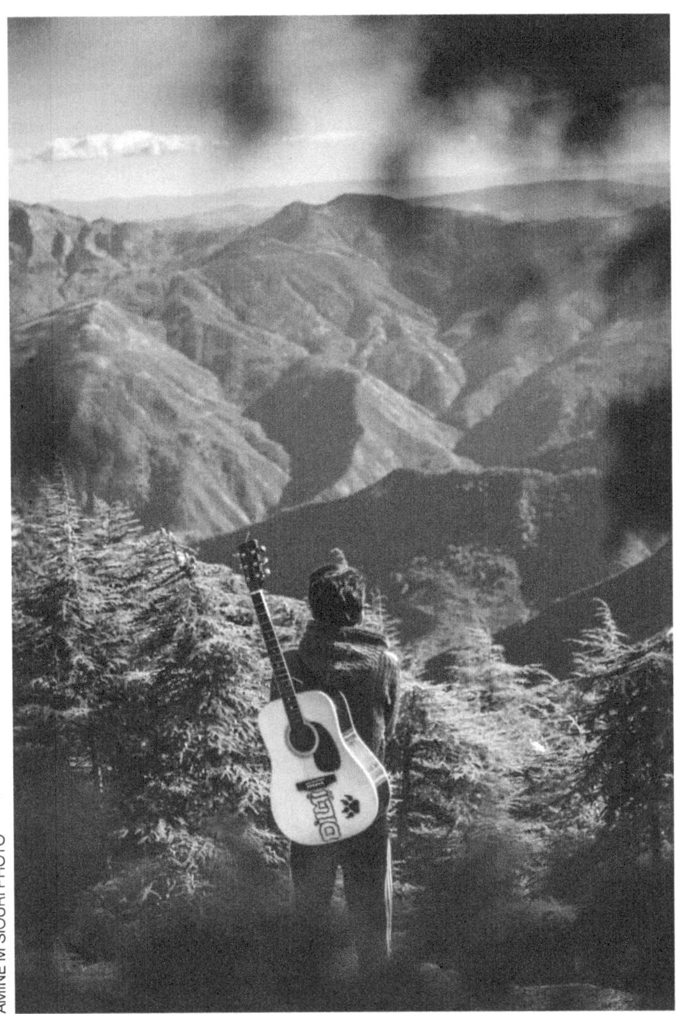

AMINE M'SIOURI PHOTO

The Benefits of Meditation

Meditation has proven immensely successful for musicians seeking to establish equilibrium, whether enduring the rigors of travel or for simply promoting relaxation, concentration, and mindfulness. There are many traditions of meditation to explore. If you're new to meditation, start by devoting a short amount of time (even 10–15 minutes) a day to sitting quietly, observing the breath, and letting persistent thoughts pass through the mind like clouds in an open sky.

Several smartphone apps offer guided meditation with soft music or natural sounds. Alternatively, you can practice in silence, focusing on each breath to release tension. One common goal of meditation is to cultivate equanimity, a gentle state where thoughts don't disturb the mind. Strengthening equanimity involves focusing gently on a homebase like breath awareness, slow counting, or a peaceful image or sound.

Establishing a regular meditation practice can be a powerful asset for managing stress and worry, common among musicians facing the pressures of the industry. Meditation promotes mental clarity, reduces stress and hypertension, and complements a practice of gratitude for music and the privilege of being a musician.

Performance Anxiety

Most guitarists have encountered anxiety or some form of stage fright at some point, which can significantly impact their performance. Studies of professional symphony orchestras indicate that up to 59% of musicians have been affected by performance anxiety in their careers.

Feeling "butterflies" before a performance is natural, and it can provide excitement and extra energy. When performance anxiety leads to marked impairment, however, it can make it difficult to concentrate and manifest through symptoms like rapid heartbeat, shaky hands, dry mouth, sweating, dizziness, and shortness of breath. These responses are triggered by cortisol, a hormone released by the adrenal glands as part of the fight-or-flight response, designed to protect us from danger.

Experiencing anxiety that feels life-threatening before a show is undesirable, but in my extensive experience as a performer and teacher, I have observed that practicing particular physical and mental exercises can replace these feelings with positive anticipation.

Mental Strategies

Take a close look at an upcoming performance and consider it from various perspectives, including that of the audience. No one attends a show hoping to see a musician fail; rather, they come to experience your artistic expression through the guitar. Many audience members make significant efforts to attend, despite fatigue or other commitments, which should reassure you that they are on your side and rooting for your success.

Preparation is irreplaceable. Investing time in practice will boost your confidence onstage. Instead of performing with doubts, trust that your thorough preparation enables you to surrender to the music and enjoy the experience of sharing music with fellow musicians and listeners. Seek inspiration from bandmates, peers, and guitar legends alike, embracing the collaborative spirit of music-making. Even as a soloist, you collaborate with your audience, which is a beautiful aspect of performing, not something to fear.

Fear often arises from lack of preparation or irrational thoughts. Negative thinking can spiral into unrealistic fears, such as catastrophic outcomes from mistakes. Some musicians find cognitive behavioral therapy (CBT) helpful in managing general anxiety issues. Onstage, there's no place for unhealthy competition, self-criticism, or imposter syndrome. Believe in your capability to share your musical gifts confidently and admirably.

Depending on the performance, you can mitigate pressure by starting with a setlist that includes pieces you know intimately and are comfortable playing. This approach ensures a strong start and allows flexibility; if one piece feels challenging in the moment, switch to another without stress. Keeping the stakes low doesn't mean playing only easy music but rather selecting well-prepared pieces that showcase your readiness through practice and visualization.

Physical Strategies

Musicians don't necessarily think of themselves as athletes, but it's important to recognize that just like athletes, we must train our bodies and adhere to essential principles of health and performance. A big part of that is making sure you are taking steps to ensure overall physical health through exercise, adequate sleep, rest, and nutrition. These will also pay dividends toward your mental well-being and your focus.

Eating foods that are high in potassium can help alleviate anxiety and tension. These foods—including bananas, leafy greens, antioxidant-rich fruits, garlic, saffron, and low-fat dairy products such as yogurt or milk—are sometimes known as natural beta blockers. Beta blockers have been shown to block the release of adrenaline, noradrenaline, and related compounds to the beta-adrenergic receptors, which can cause symptoms of high blood pressure and a racing heartbeat.

The most immediate way to physically counteract the symptoms of anxiety and stress is through breathwork. Learning various breathing techniques can have a powerful effect on your ability to relax, sharpen focus, and be present. Two common techniques include box-breathing and an ancient yogic 4-7-8 breathing strategy.

The box breathing technique involves finding a relaxed position (sitting or standing), inhaling to a slow count of four, holding the breath for four, exhaling for four, and holding again for a count of four. The 4-7-8 breath is similar in its ability to relax the body and mind: Inhale for a count of four, hold for seven, and slowly exhale to a count of eight before your next inhale. You can play with this one with the counting. For example, if you're feeling a little lethargic and need to build up some energy, try reversing the count to 8-7-4, and exhale strongly while bringing in oxygen to the slow count of eight on the inhalation. Both techniques produce wondrous and immediate physiological results that you can access anywhere, at any time.

Keeping a Journal

Many successful musicians maintain a habit of keeping a practice journal that can be used in tandem with a gig journal. One can inform the other. After a performance, for instance, you might take notes on the gig, which might include obvious mistakes, areas needing improvement, and maybe some ideas for fresher solos or chord voicings.

You can also document your sound, how gear changes worked (or didn't), anything that might have been detrimental to your performance (including unreliable gear), the flow of the set list, audience reactions, aspects of the venue, and much more. Your journal, which can be comparable to a sea captain's or pilot's logbook, can directly inform your practice journal, i.e., what you need to work on the next time you practice.

A practice journal is a great way to organize your sessions, set goals, and document progress, however gradual. For example, it can be very encouraging to look back at earlier entries and observe what you may have struggled with initially but have now mastered. There's a common phrase among musicians along the lines of, "the more you know, the more you realize you don't know," which is actually a good thing. But to avoid becoming overwhelmed, it's important to stay focused and organized, and this is where a journal can help. Some categories to document may include:

- *New songs, ideas, or concepts*
- *Works in progress*
- *Progress and work with a metronome*
- *Technical exercises*
- *Scale and arpeggio practice*
- *Triads and chord voicings*
- *Voice-leading and studies in harmony*
- *Listening, reading, and observation*
- *Tone and gear*

Visualization

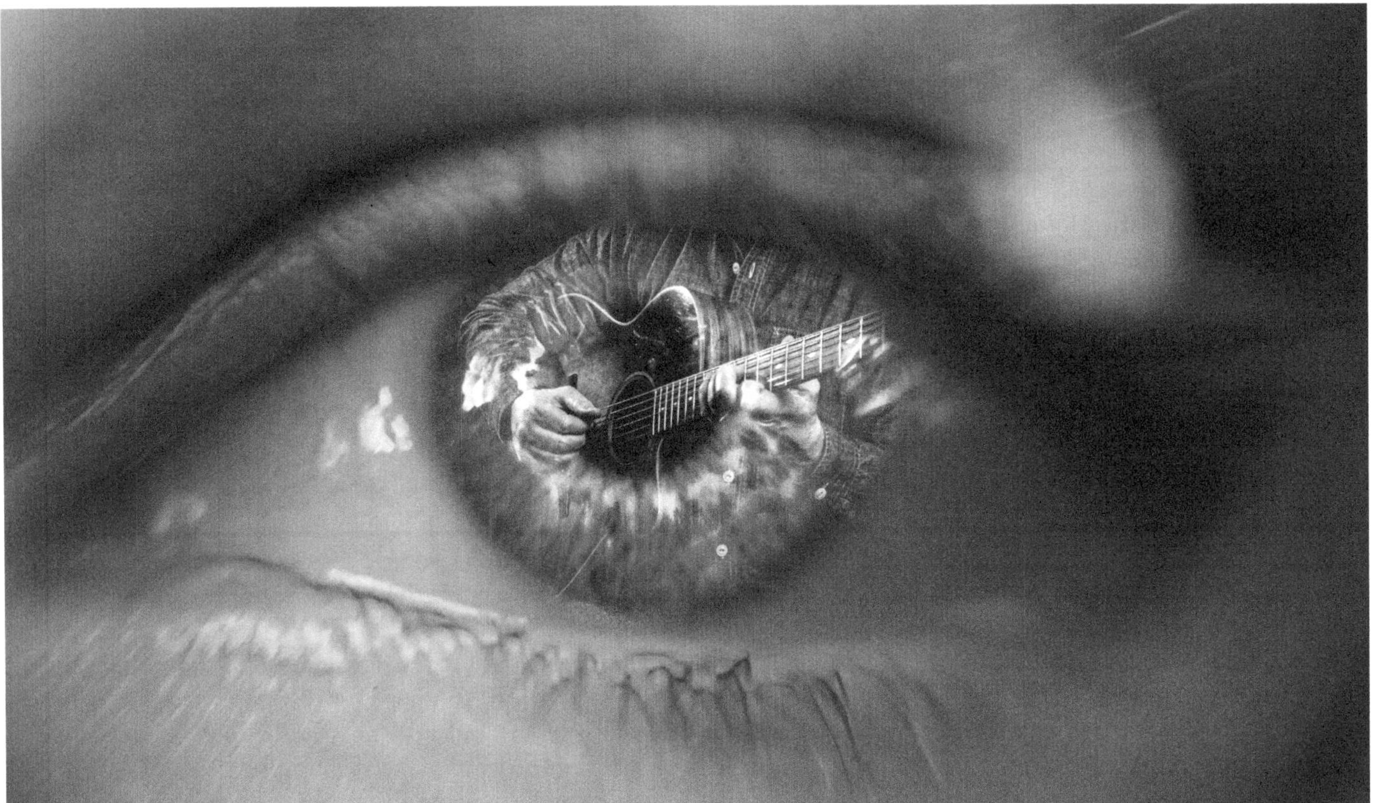

Visualization is a powerful practice that will produce immediate benefits. Even when you can't physically practice on a guitar, visualizing can improve your fretboard knowledge, rhythm, pitch and interval work, your tone, and performance.

When you are in a situation where you don't have a guitar to practice, try closing your eyes and picturing the fretboard in your mind. Visualize playing a basic scale or chord progression that is familiar. Visualize your fingers in position on the fretboard, playing individual notes or chords, and imagine what that looks and feels like. Imagine your hands crossing the strings, changing positions on the neck, etc. Neurological studies have shown that there really isn't much of a difference in the motor cortex of the brain between physically playing a scale and clearly visualizing playing one. The next time you're sitting on the couch relaxing, try visualizing scales, arpeggios, and chord voicings and progressions in your mind.

Once you become familiar with this concept, you can really utilize it to your advantage by developing your visualization skills. Try playing a melody or familiar lick, looping it over and over in your mind. As you do this, hear the pitches and rhythms with full clarity. If it helps, you can sing along, matching the pitches or verbalizing the rhythm. Hear it, see it, and feel it in your hands and body. You can also try slowing it down in your mind until you can clearly see it. We must develop dexterity in our hands through technical exercises, of course, but nine times out of ten, a mistake is usually in the mind, not the fingers. Once I have worked out a fingering in my head and can visualize playing it smoothly and perfectly, I can usually play it without any problems on the guitar. I've witnessed this phenomenon with my students, as well.

The next step is to play an entire song in your mind without stopping. Like meditation, this practice will markedly develop your ability to concentrate, and it'll improve your memorization skills. When I'm learning new music for a concert or preparing arrangements for a recording, I always spend time playing the tunes in my mind, whether it's phrasing the melody, improvising over chord changes, or playing a worked-out arrangement. I know that I'm ready for the studio or stage when I can play comfortably through the music in my mind without stopping.

I once observed a champion figure skater follow a similar practice. She positioned herself in the middle of an ice rink, and as her program music played, she sat without moving and visualized her entire routine, right down to the second, for about five and a half minutes. Visualizing in this way not only strengthens the connection between the mind and body, but it also avoids overtaxing the body by repeatedly running a routine. Award-winning classical guitarist and educator William Kanengiser offers, "If you can see it in your mind, you can do it with your fingers. Always be able to play through a piece from beginning to end in your mind before stepping onstage."

Finally, you can use the practice and skill of visualization to work on your sound, compositional style, musical identity, and stage presence. Try envisioning the tone of some of your favorite guitarists in your imagination. Chances are, if you've listened to them deeply, you can easily hear their sound in your head. Now try to hear your tone. What does it sound like? Can you hear it clearly? What do you sound like? How does it compare to your influences? If it's not overtly clear, try to analyze some aspects of the sound of your influences.

Instead of their gear, think about how your influences produce tone through their picking techniques, use of rhythm and phrasing, and slurring through hammer-ons, slides, and pull-offs. Notice whether their tone is bright or dark. Pay attention to their awareness of dynamics and their overall touch on the guitar. Once you break these down, you can begin to apply what you like to your concept of sound; only then can you play guitar and match the sound you hear in your mind.

You can try this same visualization practice with writing music. Many musicians will start with a groove, beat, or singing a melodic phrase. Once you get it going, write your idea down or record yourself singing it on your phone. While it's great to write music with the guitar, it can also be very satisfying and organic to compose away from the guitar and just from your mind.

You can also visualize what you want to look like on stage and how this aesthetic relates to your sound. In the same way you can hear the tone of your favorite players in your head, you can clearly imagine seeing what they look like when performing. This practice can also help develop confidence and mitigate performance anxiety. As an exercise, picture yourself walking on stage with total confidence. You look great, you have done everything necessary to prepare for this show, and now you're ready to deliver an incredible performance.

Picture yourself playing flawlessly through your set and connecting with the audience. You can imagine, in between songs perhaps, telling stories about the pieces or connecting with the audience through humor. The point is that you are envisioning a successful performance in detail, and in doing so, you are setting yourself up for success. After you've spent enough time practicing in your mind, it's bound to happen—just like practicing a scale over and over.

Concentration and Memorization

Regardless of whether they typically play music by ear or by reading sheet music, most guitarists agree that they perform better and have a much deeper connection to the music if it's memorized. By taking your eyes off the page, you can concentrate on tone, phrasing, dynamics, emotion, and techniques in focused detail.

Researchers have described three principal functions when memorizing music: aural, visual, and kinesthetic. Aural memory allows the guitarist to hear a melody or chord progression internally, while visual memory consists of connecting notes on the page to fingerings and recognizing rhythms, melodic patterns, and chord shapes. Kinesthetic memory (also known as finger or tactile memory) is developed and accessed through repeated muscle movements by synchronizing fretting and picking between the two hands and being able to replicate those movements away from the guitar.

When learning and memorizing a piece of music, it's important to start with an overview of structure and form, followed by a harmonic analysis. What is the form of the song? Where are the repeats? How many measures are in each section? Then focus on the harmony through analytical methods such as traditional Roman numeral harmonic analysis or the Nashville number system. Knowledge of music theory and extensive experience studying and playing music can help immensely in the process of memorizing because you'll have something to relate to and draw upon similarities with other pieces.

If you're memorizing written music, try reading through the entire piece and imagine playing it on the guitar. Picture the fingerings, changes in position and strings, picking patterns, etc. Several research studies have shown the advantages of chunking, or breaking a large piece of music down into smaller sections that are easy to internalize through repetition.

Finally, you can develop both your concentration and skill with memorization by singing/approximating the melody while visualizing the harmony or chords and fretboard; observing changes in tempo, time, or dynamics; transitions to new sections; and experiencing every moment of the song before playing it on the guitar. You will notice a visceral experience when you combine all these visualization techniques prior to playing it on the guitar, as well as experience a comfortable ease and natural flow as a result of memorizing the music in this way.

CHAPTER FIVE

The Spirit of a Musician

A major component of health and wellness for guitarists is to focus on and keep close to heart and mind all the positive benefits of playing an instrument and living a life enriched by music. Many guitarists consider their journey in music—whether consciously or subconsciously—no less than a spiritual commitment. Indeed, dedication to a lifelong musical practice of excellence is akin to a spiritual practice, one that is often and affirmatively rooted in gratitude and fortitude.

Sometimes, the challenges of making a living as a professional guitarist in the modern world can seem overwhelming.

But the insatiable desire to keep going, to improve our playing and enrich our lives, is what is important and sustainable. I like to think of the indomitable spirit of musicians: Our dedicated practice of self-improvement and offering beauty to the world is a never-ending continuum that connects us to many generations of musicians, both past and future. Learning how to connect with gratitude, appreciation, optimism, creativity, and reflection can help to keep the flame burning for many years to come.

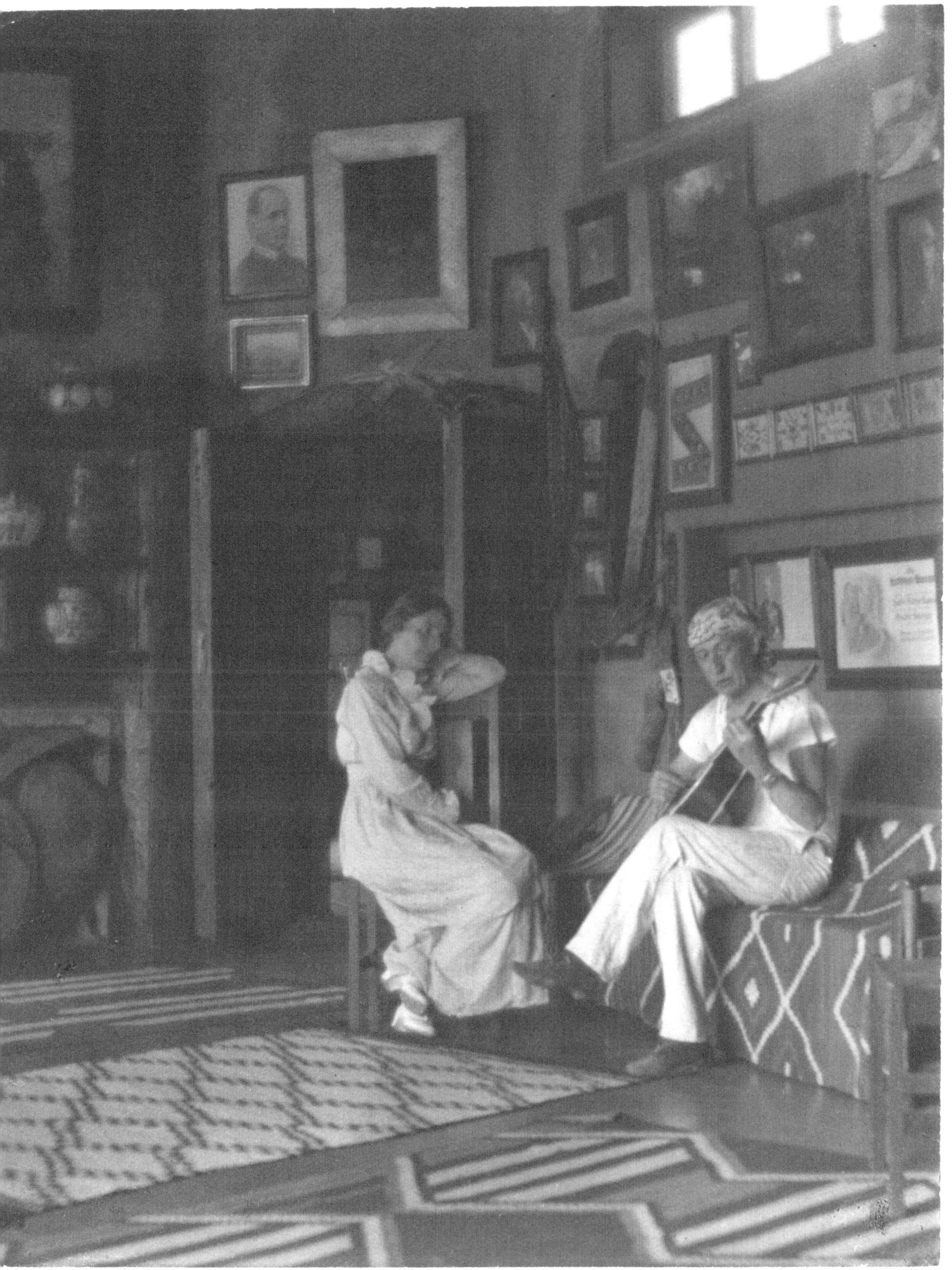

LOUIS FLECKENSTEI PHOTO

Prelude No. 5

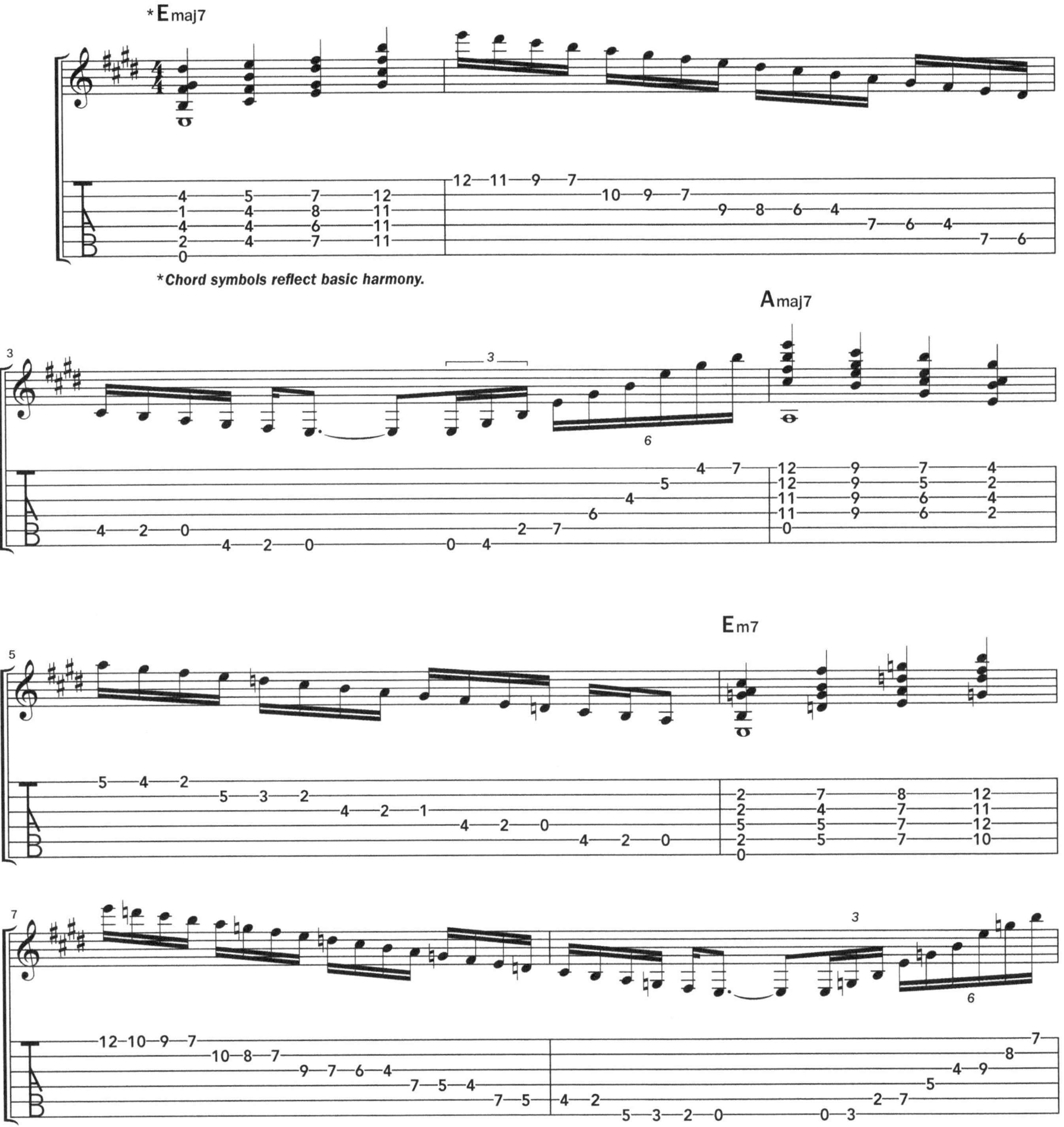

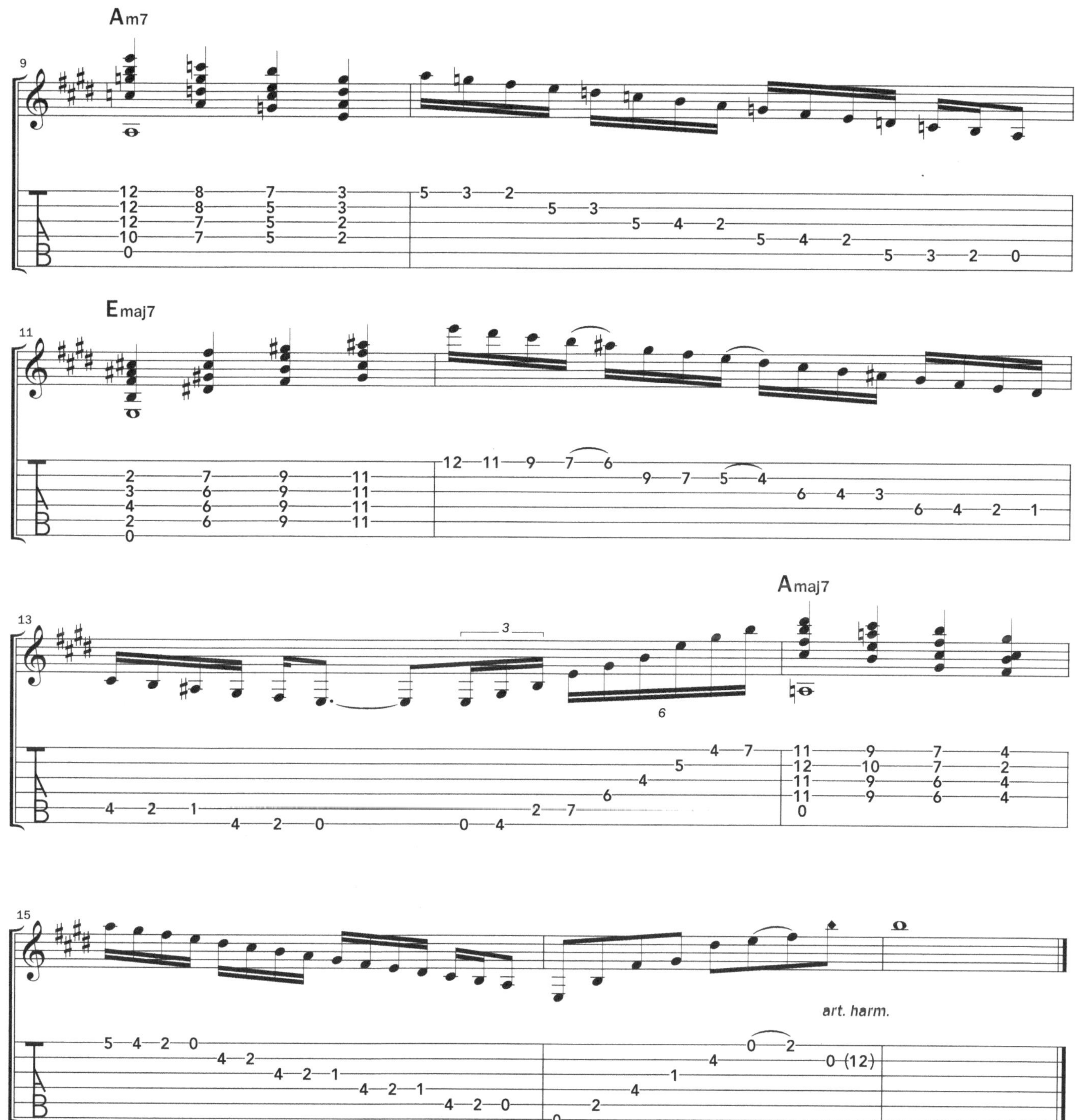
Am7
Emaj7
Amaj7
art. harm.

The Practice of Gratitude and Looking Deeply

Vietnamese Zen Buddhist monk Thich Nhat Hanh was an influential figure all over the world through his many writings, dharma talks, retreats, and deep reflection on adapting ancient wisdom and teachings for modern society. His books, including the seminal *Being Peace* and *Touching Peace*, feature many different methods and techniques to develop and practice gratitude, especially in the midst of challenging times.

One technique is to look deeply at a regular activity, one that may even be taken for granted, such as drinking tea. As an avid coffee enthusiast, I use this example with my students, but you can imagine tea or any type of food. Instead of mindlessly drinking a cup of coffee, recognize the numerous steps that ultimately brought that cup of coffee to you: How the coffee trees were planted and carefully cultivated at just the right altitude and in the right climate, how the coffee cherries were delicately picked at just the right time, and how they were then dried and hulled to produce the green beans, which were shipped to master roasters who have dedicated their lives to learning, practicing, and mastering the art of roasting and tasting. After traveling many miles from different continents and passing through many expert and caring hands, the beans arrive ready for meticulous grinding and brewing into a cup of coffee, which ultimately ends up in your hands to help you conquer the morning and achieve your goals.

Once I started this practice, I never again took drinking coffee for granted. Recognizing the work that goes into creating a cup of coffee, often shared with family, good friends, and musical colleagues, gave me perspective and a profound sense of gratitude.

I also apply this practice to my instruments. Think about it: For many years, the guitars you own were trees in places such as Africa, Brazil, India, the Pacific Northwest, Southeastern Asia, and New England. I think about the dedicated adventurers who harvested, salvaged, and transported the wood. I think of the experts who recognize the perfect wood for soundboards; the selection and purchase by luthiers who have dedicated their lives to the art of guitar building; the incredible forethought and intense manual labor that goes into sawing, shaping, and bending the sides of the wood, as well as the tuning of the top and placement of bracing—all things that have taken years of trial and error to master. I reflect on the careful selection of materials, electronics, binding, purfling, aesthetic applications, inlays, as well as other organic materials used such as bone and abalone.

I think of all the great minds and hands that created the guitars we love to play, which will in turn enrich the lives of others through music. It's incredible! I love to admire my guitars, and I deeply appreciate their origin as trees, often from the other side of the globe, as well as the work that went into creating them.

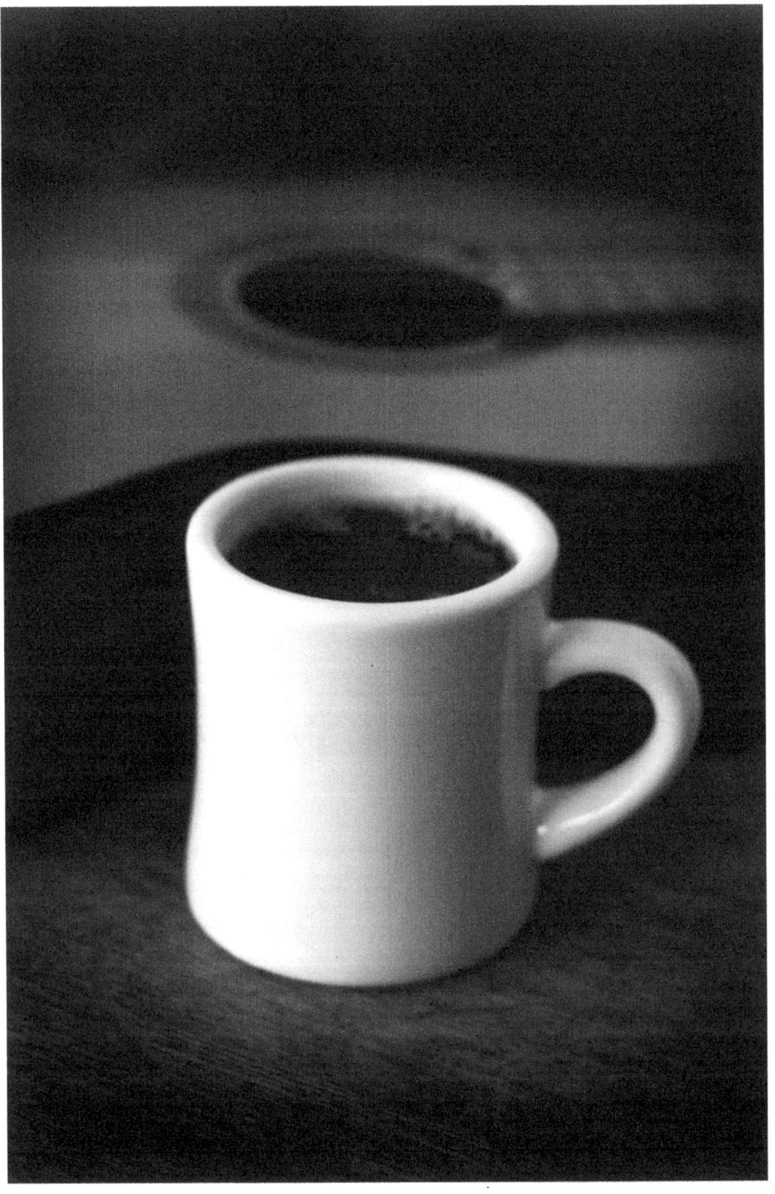

“

The whole cosmos has come together to create you. You carry the whole cosmos inside you. That is why to accept yourself and to love yourself is an expression of gratitude.”

—Thich Nhat Hanh

Japanese Concepts

The ongoing practice of music requires significant dedication, and musicians often turn to philosophical and spiritual traditions for inspiration. There are several Japanese concepts—at once ancient and modern—that can inform our practice as guitarists. Any concept that helps inspire, alleviate anxiousness, or renew with a fresh perspective is certainly worth looking at. In my experience, the following concepts can be very helpful when applied to a life and practice in music.

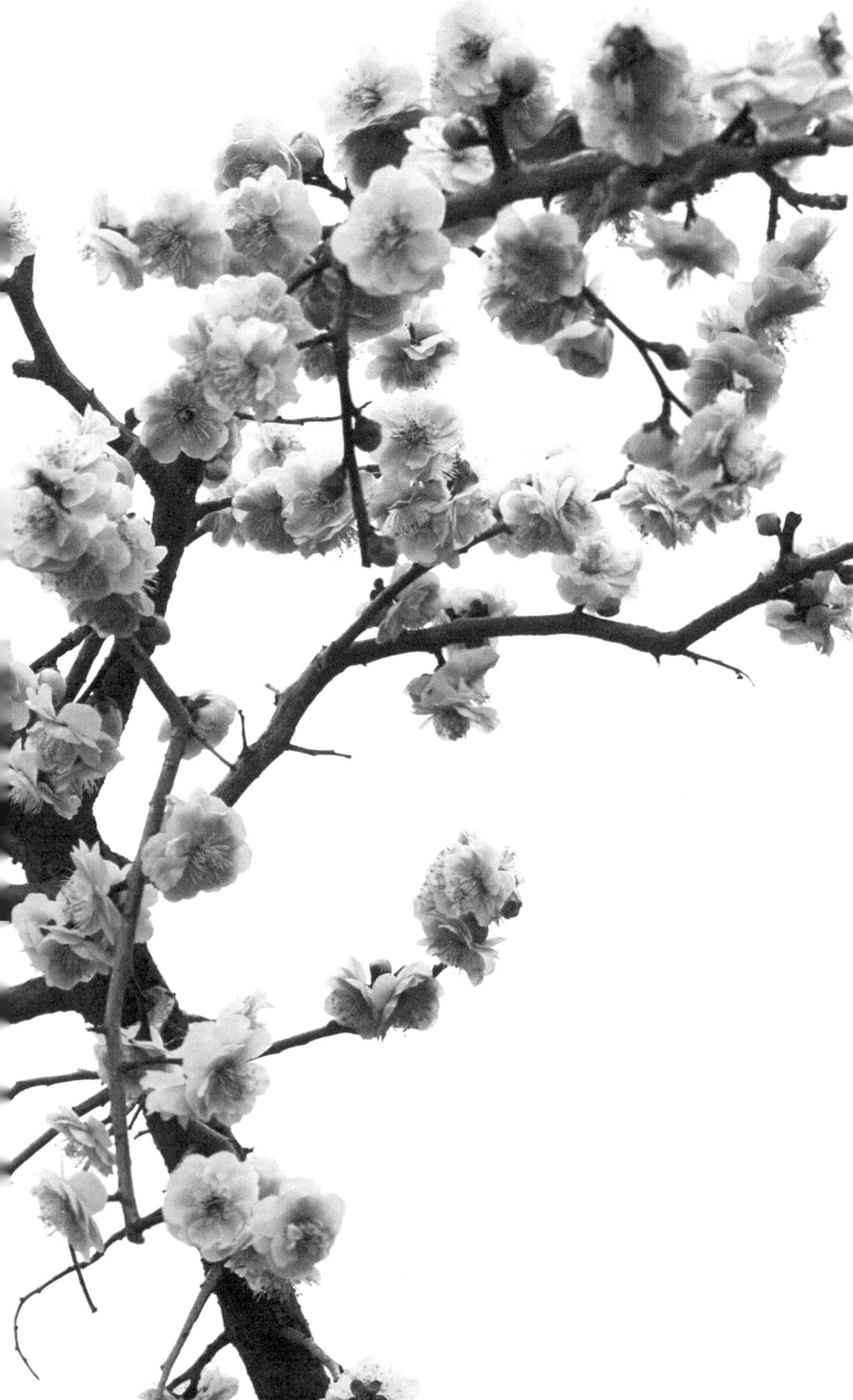

Ikigai

Iki roughly translates to "life" or "alive," while *gai* translates to "benefit" or "worth." *Ikigai* is a term commonly considered to embody one's purpose in life—literally, a reason for living. Many guitarists, especially professionals, can identify with this concept. Although there are so many challenges that face musicians—societal bias, financial hardship, physical and psychological strain—professional guitarists often say they had no choice but to dedicate their lives to music, regardless of the outcome. The concept of ikigai is just as important for non-professional guitarists. Contemporary psychologists often cite "the reason for getting out of bed every day" as an important indicator of wellness and a sense of purpose.

Ikigai can also be considered an intersection of ideas when deciding what it is you love to do, developing your skills, figuring out how to make a living, and aligning with what the world needs (and the world will always need music and the arts). Ikigai can describe the feeling of accomplishment and deep satisfaction of pursuing a passion; according to psychologist Katsuya Inoue, ikigai can also embody objects that bring meaning to life. This concept resonates with guitarists who find considerable joy in their instruments and in playing music, whether it's for their own enjoyment or for public performance. To this end, it can be extremely satisfying to set performance goals in your community, whether playing in a local coffee house, wine bar, community center, or house of worship.

Dedicating oneself to music is a noble endeavor, and many people find renewed inspiration in learning, relearning, or improving their abilities. This often happens when guitarists who may have had a career outside of music reach retirement age and can fully dedicate their time to attain their goals in music and the guitar. I've witnessed incredible improvement among many of my students who were finally able to devote time to playing guitar as retirees, and their lives were richly rewarded. But recognizing a deep sense of purpose and identity through playing music is important for anyone at any stage in their life or career.

Kaizen

Applying the principles of kaizen, "good change," can be powerfully beneficial to the practice and study of guitar. In her book, *Kaizen: The Japanese Method for Transforming Habits One Small Step at a Time*, Sarah Harvey offers numerous examples of integrating kaizen into daily life. I have found the following examples helpful for guitarists.

Small Changes Lead to Continual Improvement

Steady progress is built upon changes that are easy to adapt to. This might include learning new scales, chord forms, or songs just one piece at a time. For example, you might spend an entire practice session focusing on the verse or one part of a song, and then work on the next part or chorus the following day or even the following week. If you spend enough time patiently working on one part and really dig in, by the time you move on, that first part will be internalized, and you won't have to spend time relearning it.

Consistency is Key

Whenever possible, get into a consistent guitar routine that makes sense with your personal life and work schedules. It's much better to practice every day for a short amount of time than once or twice a week for longer periods. If you can get in some time every morning and/or later in the day, you'll notice significant improvements. Practicing consistently trains your mind and your hands, solves musical and technical problems, and builds a solid foundation of technique.

Focus on the Process

Of course, we want to focus on our goals, which might include playing songs, being able to improvise, and creating inventive rhythm parts. But if you can home in on the process of learning, you'll learn on a deeper level and enjoy the time spent doing the work. Studies have shown that when we are having fun—notice the word "play"—we learn more efficiently. Surrender the results, enjoy the process at whatever stage you're currently in, and have faith that through consistent work, you will achieve your guitar goals.

Embrace Failure

Don't beat yourself up if you make mistakes on the gig, in the studio, or in the practice room. Simply observe the problem and get to the root of the issue by working on it slowly and methodically. This is where a practice journal can come in handy. For instance, after a gig, you might write down some of the things that went wrong or weren't quite up to par. The next time you sit down to practice, all these things will be in your journal and ready for work. Failure can be a great motivator—as long as you don't let it haunt you. Instead, commit to patiently working on whatever it is, gradually ensuring that it won't ever be an issue again.

Seek Feedback and Create a Supportive Environment

Establishing a musical community is one of the best ways to improve your musicianship. It's also a great way to make music with trusted friends and/or teachers. Many songwriters, for example, belong to a writing community (online or in person) with whom they share works in progress, holding each other accountable to timelines. Nothing can motivate quite like a deadline! There are similar jazz guitar study groups where members all learn the same standard and work through different ways of interpreting, comping, and improvising on it. We all know that practicing can be solitary, and sometimes that's a good thing. But if you can get together with a friend or even start a practice group, you will notice palpable strides in your development, and you'll have a good time while you're at it!

> *"If you want to have a good harvest, the most important thing is to make the soil rich and cultivate it well."*
>
> —Shunryu Suzuki

"I have a theory that the moment one gives close attention to anything, even a blade of grass, it becomes a mysterious, awesome, indescribably magnificent world in itself. I have tried this experiment a thousand times and I have never been disappointed. The more I look at a thing, the more I see in it, and the more I see in it, the more I want to see. It is like peeling an onion. There is always another layer, and another, and another. And each layer is more beautiful than the last.

This is the way I look at the world. I don't see it as a collection of objects, but as a vast and mysterious organism. I see the beauty in the smallest things, and I find wonder in the most ordinary events. I am always looking for the hidden meaning, the secret message. I am always trying to understand the mystery of life. I know that I will never understand everything, but that doesn't stop me from trying. I am content to live in the mystery, to be surrounded by the unknown. I am content to be a seeker, a pilgrim, a traveler on the road to nowhere."

—Henry Miller

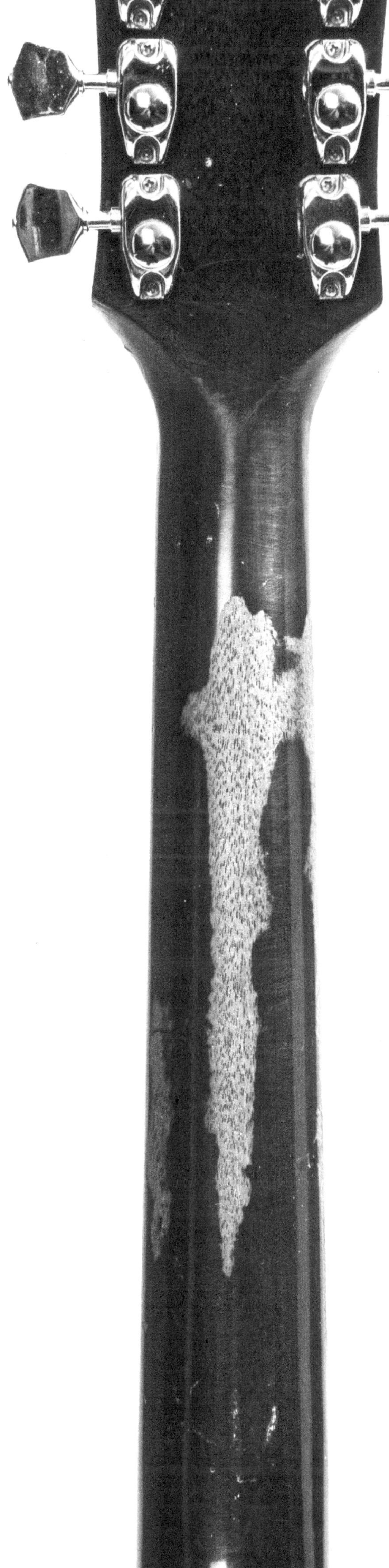

Celebrate Your Progress

Give credit where credit is due. If that means learning new repertoire, being able to play new things effortlessly, coming up with creative ideas and music, playing in public, etc., then by all means, celebrate! Again, this is where a practice/gig journal can help you out. You might find yourself looking back at the challenges from last week, month, or year and be surprised at what you struggled with in the practice room. This observation will help your confidence and mindset time and time again. Sometimes, it's not easy to recognize progress when you're in the middle of a challenging situation, but when you can look at something with the benefit of hindsight, you'll often be amazed at the progress you've made. Just think about how forming basic open position and barre chords—or anything else you struggled with in the beginning—once seemed overwhelming. It's always a good time to celebrate the wins!

Wabi-sabi

This term describes a concept that is prevalent throughout Japanese society yet is ineffable or difficult at best to express in words. Essentially, it is an aesthetic concept that finds beauty in imperfection. It involves recognizing the impermanence of things and therefore finding peace and joy within the inconsistencies of life.

Wabi-sabi can offer a profoundly positive influence on musical practice. By releasing the idea of perfection in the studio or on stage and surrendering to the moment, for instance, guitarists can tap into a greater sense of flow, which often results in more inspired and authentic music. Embracing imperfection and the freedom of spontaneity can yield tremendous benefits to your music, as well as a steady sense of satisfaction. Recognizing the fragility of life can help you develop patience and acceptance, which leads to focusing on the best version of oneself and avoiding the traps of competition rooted in self-doubt.

Shinrin-yoku

Shinrin-yoku, "forest bathing," is a Japanese concept that is gaining popularity in the Western world as more and more scientific studies show the benefits of spending time in nature—not necessarily hiking or sport, but rather simply enjoying elements that stimulate the senses: the scent of fir, pine, and rain in the woods; the sight of sunlight streaming through the trees; the sound of leaves crackling and crunching, as well as the songs of birds, insects, and wildlife. Shinrin-yoku can bring peace and clarity that will lift your guitar playing to higher levels.

Finding Inspiration

Inspiration can come from many different sources, from getting outside and spending time in nature, visiting a new place or city, or checking out an art gallery or museum to watching a movie or reading a good book. Of course, it can also come from listening to inspired music—especially live music. One of the reasons musicians in concentrated scenes such as New York City or Nashville stay connected is that they regularly attend performances by their contemporaries. Going to inspiring shows and then performing your own is truly a reciprocal experience. Get into the habit of going to see local music regularly, and get to know the best musicians. It's always a good idea to have great players to draw from when you're looking for other musicians to play with.

Another source of inspiration is simply listening to your favorite guitarists and learning about them and their music. Learning the stories behind your go-to records or discovering how your favorite artists stay inspired, write songs, and come up with new tunings and techniques can yield an incredible amount of inspiration and energy.

Of course, sometimes it can be important to take a break from practicing—and even from listening to music for a little while—to find inspiration. Silence and introspection can also be inspiring and refreshing, especially after an intense musical period.

The concept of change can be difficult to embrace, but change itself can be inspiring. Switching up your routine—playing different guitars, trying new gear, practicing new things and learning new music, even taking a trip to another city to hear live music and experience the sights and sounds—can recharge your spirit.

Finally, be sure to recognize your uniqueness. There will only ever be one of you in this world, and it's important to trust your own intuition and musical direction, especially when building your own musical identity. Being aware of what makes you unique, accepting and then cultivating your unique attributes will provide a deeply organic comfort.

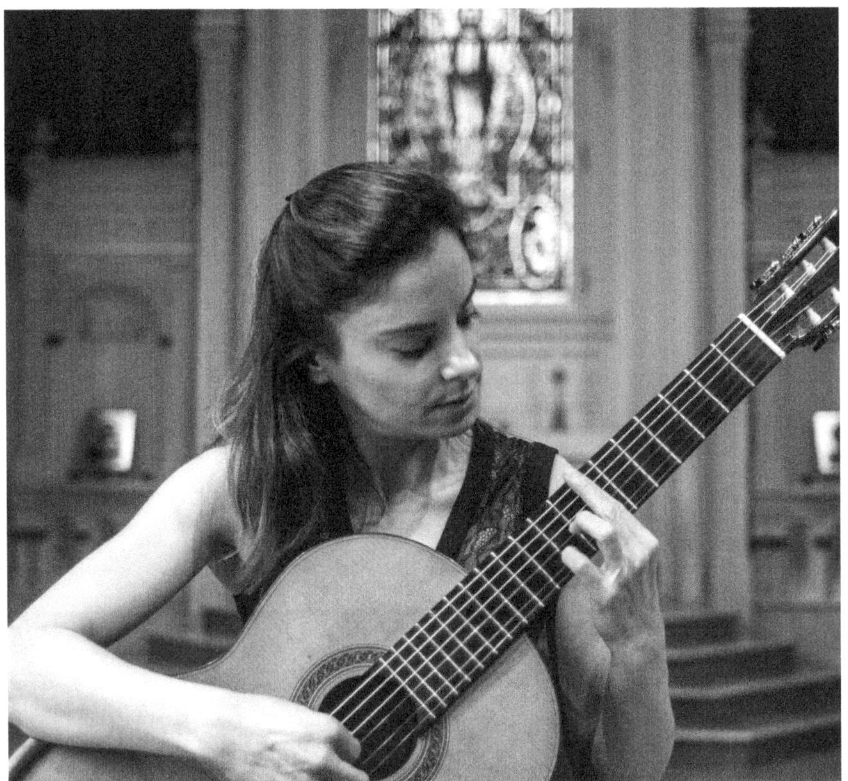

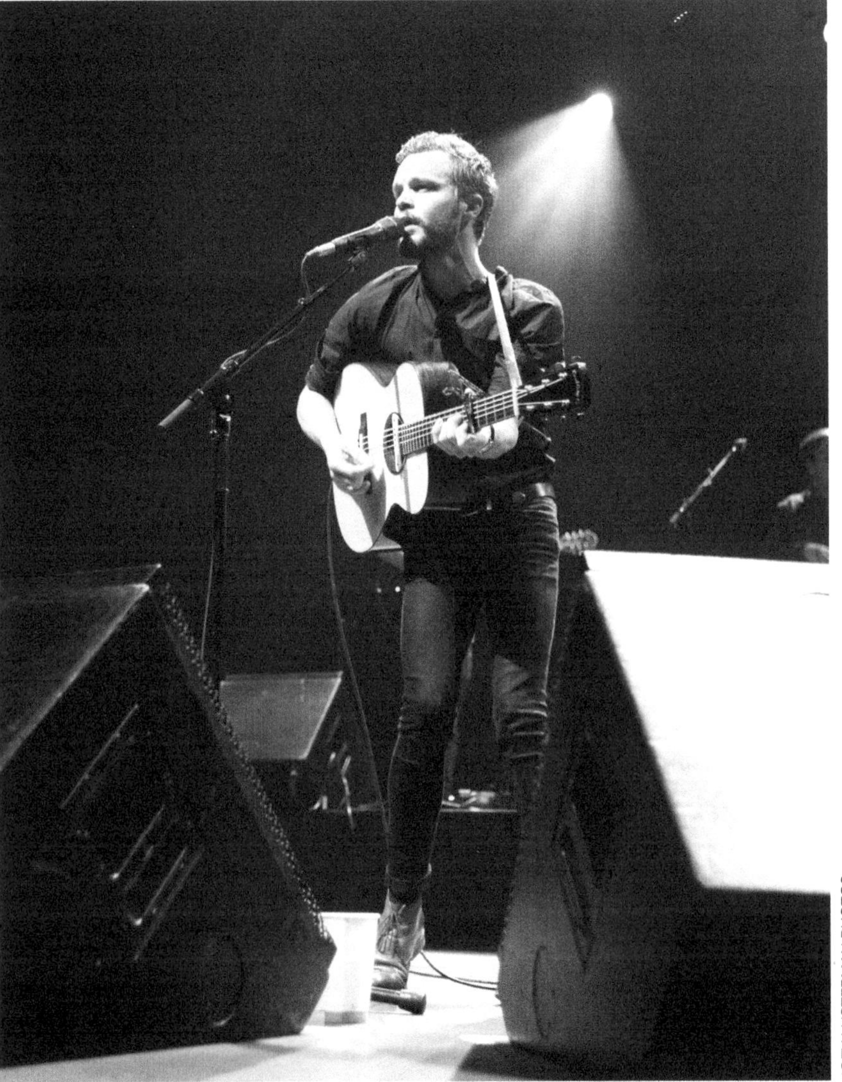

JOEY LUSTERMAN PHOTOS

Ana Vidovic at St. Mark's Church and The Tallest Man on Earth at the Fox Theater

“

I have a firm belief in this now, not only in terms of my own experience, but in knowing the experiences of other people. When you follow your bliss, and by bliss I mean the deep sense of being in it, and doing what the push is out of your own existence—it may not be fun, but it's your bliss and there's bliss behind pain, too...You follow that and doors will open where there were no doors before, where you would not have thought there'd be doors, and where there wouldn't be a door for anybody else.”

—Joseph Campbell

CHAPTER SIX

Building a Solid Foundation of Technique

One of the most elusive aspects of playing guitar involves the development of solid technique, particularly speed. Indeed, it seems that every style requires a certain level of technical ability to play the repertoire convincingly.

But it's also important to look at the larger picture. Technique represents the embodiment of your relationship with the guitar, which includes your own personal sound, concept, style, dynamics, good tone, and rhythmic acuity, as well as dexterity and speed.

After all, consider that the Spanish phrase *tocar la guitarra* means "touch the guitar."

Your technique is based on your touch, which is informed by your approach, musical concepts, and the sounds you hear in your head. Therefore, we can work on developing our touch and technical ability to allow for any style we wish to play, particularly musical styles that may involve improvisation, which require a quick reaction time and solid command of the fretboard.

In this chapter, we will explore several ways to develop a solid understanding and foundation of technique that suits your own playing style while developing strength, fluidity, and independence in the fretting hand and working through numerous picking and fingerstyle approaches in exercises and études.

Prelude No. 6

G6/9
F6/9
Fmaj9
5
E♭maj9
D9sus4
A♭m7
Gm9
9
Bm11
Cm11
Bm11/E
Cm11
E9sus4
F9sus4
Amaj7
F♯m11

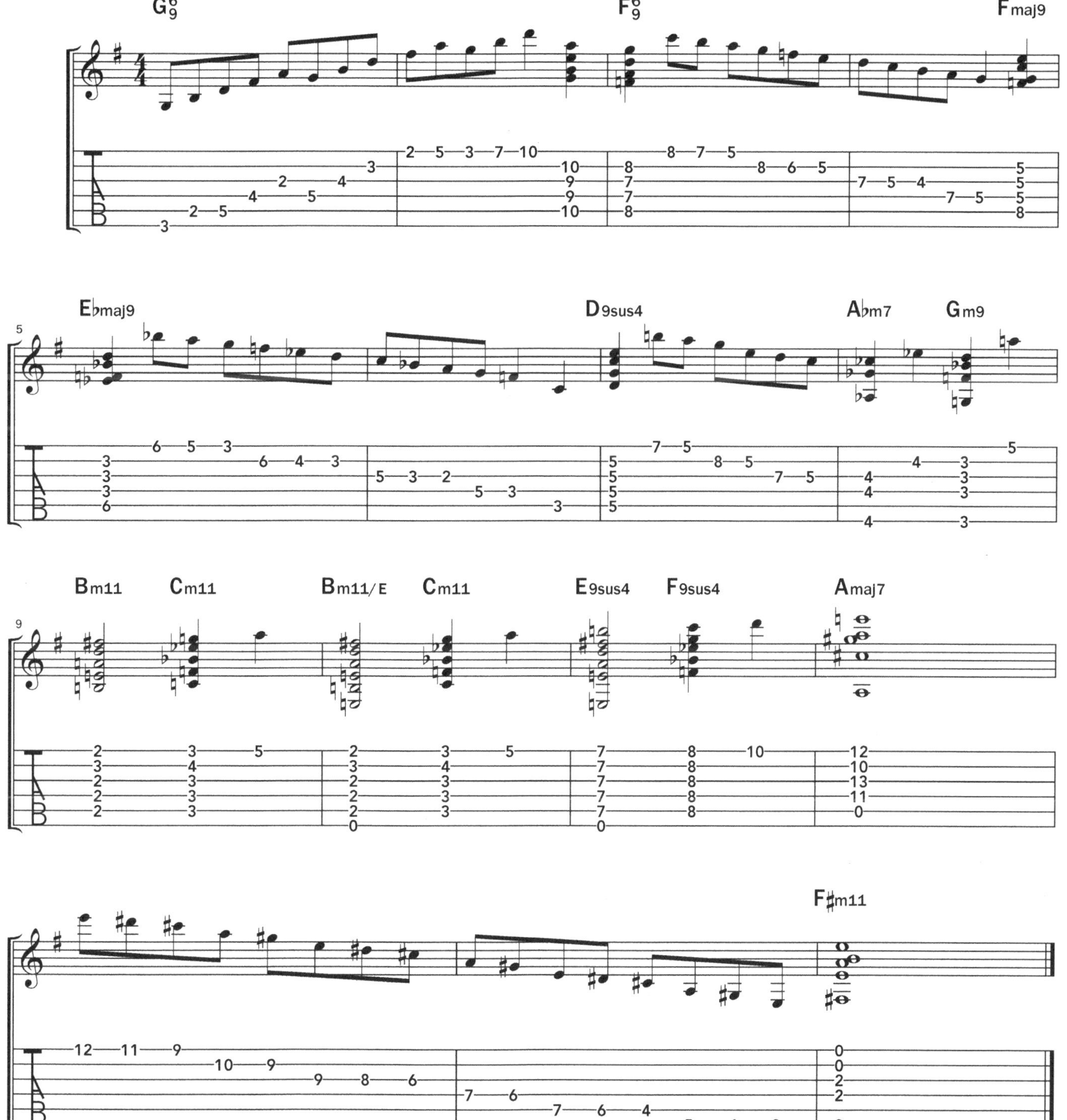

Dial in the Details, Unwind the Mind

General synonyms for technique include skill, style, routine, and approach, all ideas we can incorporate as we practice with the goal of delivery in sound. We are attracted to our favorite musicians and music primarily because of the sound. With that in mind, after you have briefly stretched your hands and body, you can start a practice session with simple exercises emphasizing good tone production. This will require an intense focus on your sound, considering and creating a keen self-awareness of the following factors that most directly affect and influence your tone.

Flatpicking

- The size, thickness, and material of your pick
- The side of the pick you use
- The angle of the pick as it connects to the string (e.g. perpendicular, at an angle, parallel)
- Your dynamic range (i.e. how loud/soft you can play, and your attack under different circumstances, e.g. with a band, singer, playing solo, etc.)

Fingerstyle

- Whether or not you use nails
- If you use nails, the length, shape, and material (natural nail, acrylic)
- The posture of the hand and wrist, and the velocity of individual fingers

Fretting Hand

- Maintaining a relaxed neutral arc ("classical") position, with the thumb lightly flexed at the back center of the neck to support finger movement
- Strong connection to the fretboard with the fingertips, without pressing too hard, staying on the wood and off the frets to avoid buzzing and ensure a solid, consistent tone

Once you establish a basic framework of tone production, you can experiment with other acoustic tonal factors such as string types, gauges, and materials, followed by tonewood types and guitar body/construction. These will be followed by electronic considerations such as pickups, microphones, and amplification, but the core of your tone starts in your ears, with your hands largely responsible for your unique sound.

Many instrumentalists, including violinists, cellists, and saxophonists, start practice sessions with long tones. This is not often the case with guitarists, perhaps because we don't have to worry about intonation or breathing, as other instrumentalists do; we also have inherently limited sustain. However, it's a good idea to start by playing slow, long tones, allowing each note to bloom to its fullest potential.

Better yet, record yourself and listen to the beginning (pick/finger attack), middle (note pitch, tone, bloom/sustain), and end (decay) of each note. By paying close attention, you will also develop the ability to concentrate, which is like a muscle. As a bonus, your focus will be strictly on your guitar tone and not distracted by the goings-on of the day.

Let's look at **Examples 1–2c**. These figures illustrate playing long tones, free of rhythm or time, using one-, two-, and three-note structures. The point is to focus on the sound, connecting your hands, ears, and guitar. When thinking strictly of tone production, many guitarists prefer using downstrokes, which are generally stronger and easier to play. If you do play more than one note, focus on the clarity and evenness of every single note.

One technique to try in these examples is using the pick to drag into the next adjacent string. When playing the first two bars of Ex. 1, drag the pick down through the D and G strings, using the B string as a wall to stop the pick motion. For the next two bars, use a downstroke for the notes on the G and B strings, using the high E to stop the pick.

Conversely, fingerstyle players can create

this rest stroke effect by plucking the index or middle finger from the top note down, ultimately resting up into the A string for the first two bars, and the D string for measures 3–4. **Example 3** shows G major triads moving across the fretboard in different inversions, positions, and string sets. While the example is notated with quarter notes, don't worry about playing these in strict tempo. The point is to warm up the hands and listen to your sound intently. **Example 4** moves through different triad types, all using the same string set moving up and down the fretboard horizontally.

It's important to note that all the examples in this chapter may be played (in fact, it's strongly encouraged) both with a pick and fingerstyle.

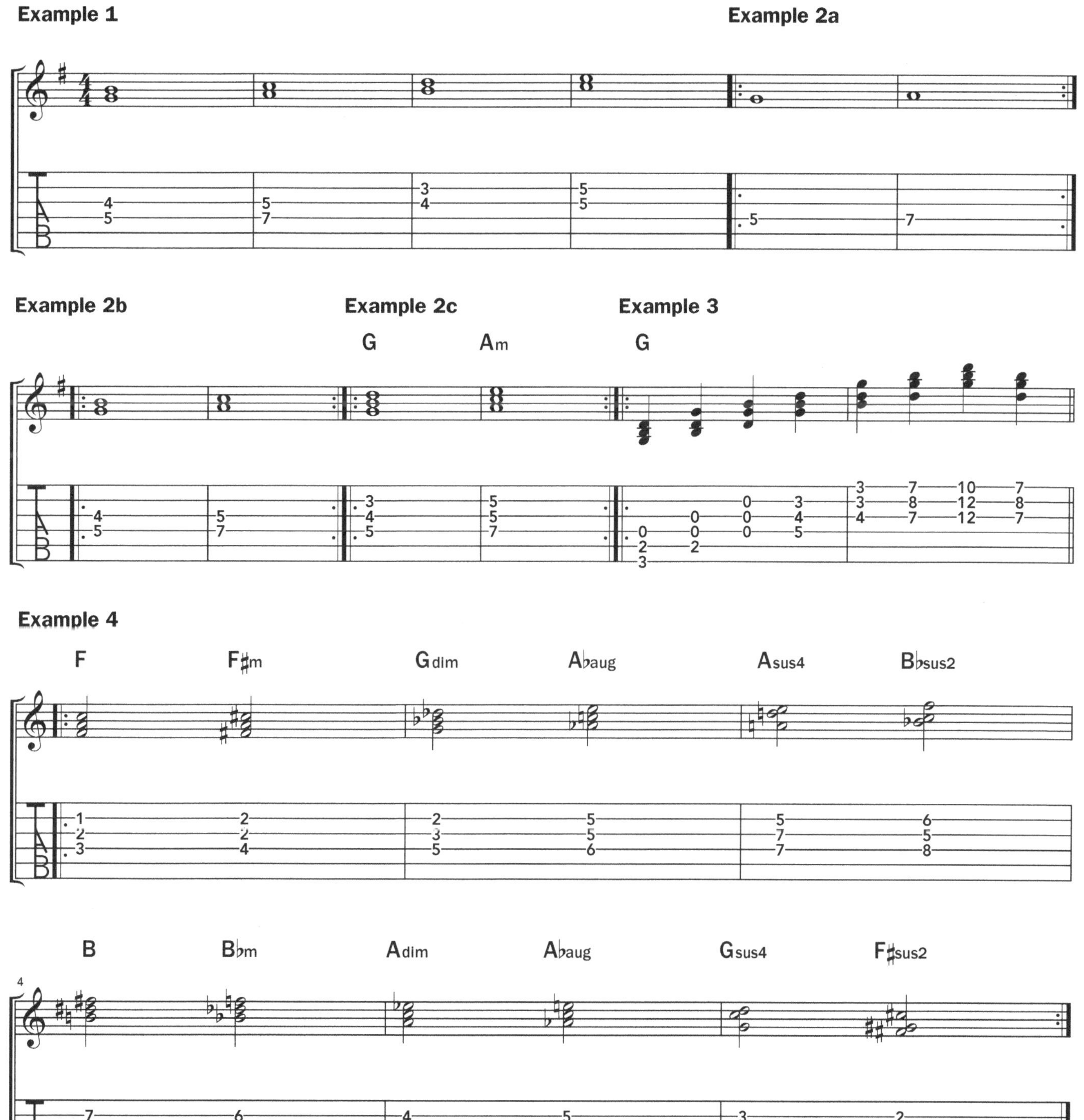

Exploring Dynamics, Articulation, and Rhythm

Now let's play through **Example 5**, which shows a common fingering for an E major scale (E F# G# A B C# D#) in fourth position. Instead of just running the scale ascending and descending, let's explore our dynamic range. Try recording this example three times. First, play as softly as you can—like a whisper, barely audible—while still aiming for a solid tone and connection to the strings. Next, play it as loudly as you can without completely sacrificing the tone (e.g., avoiding buzzing or distortion). Finally, start softly and gradually crescendo so that the notes on the high E string are the loudest, then gradually decrease the volume as you descend the scale. Imagine that someone else is gradually turning a giant volume knob up and then down while you're playing through the scale. That's the effect you want to create in this exercise.

Examples 6 and **7** focus on developing control and articulation by accenting different notes. Both examples portray a one-octave C major scale (C D E F G A B) with different notes to accent—regardless of whether it's a down- or up-stroke (or i-m if playing fingerstyle). Each measure of Ex. 6 features one pitch in the scale to accent or to play significantly louder than the others. In the first two bars, accent all C notes; in the following bars, accent the D and E, respectively. You can gradually work through the entire scale, accenting one note at a time in succession, always using alternate picking (or alternating i-m).

It's challenging because the accented notes alternate between downstrokes (stronger) and upstrokes (weaker). However, strive to make them both equally strong, and try to keep the unaccented notes consistent

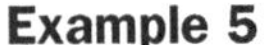

Example 5

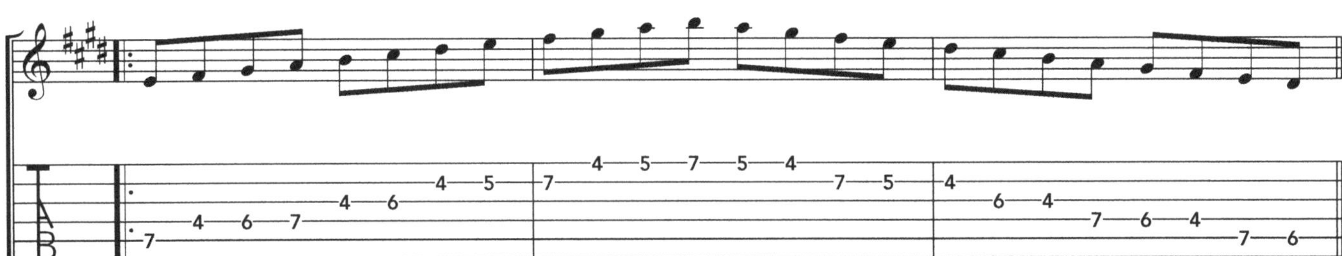

Example 6

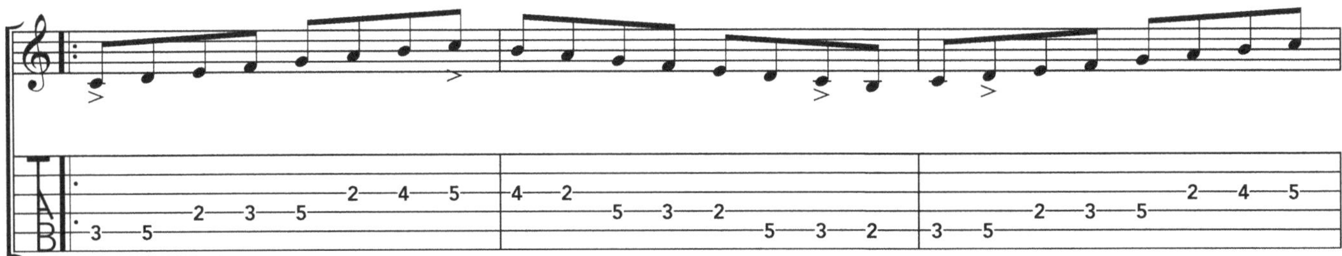

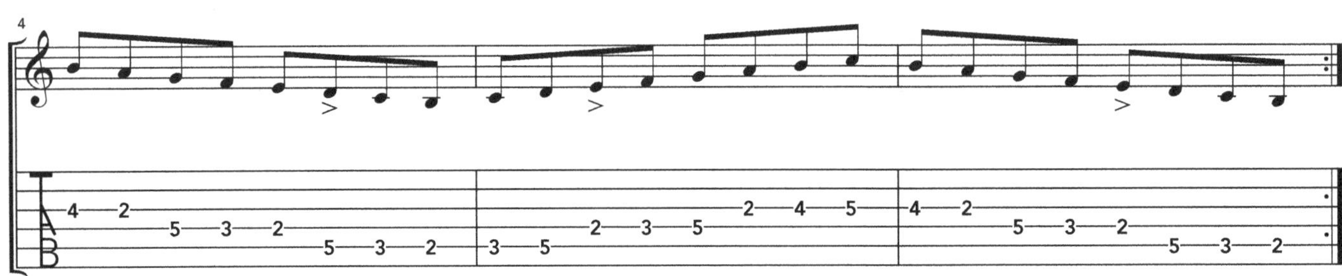

in volume. Again, thinking of the giant volume knob, set your unaccented notes at a certain volume and imagine the accented pitches quickly spiking in volume. Ex. 7 expands on this concept by accenting two pitches (F and C) within the span of one measure. To mix things up, try randomly picking any two notes within the scale to accent while practicing this major scale fingering.

Now let's practice some exercises that will develop your rhythmic acuity. **Examples 8a–f** work through a melodic fragment in G major, using a consistent fingering pattern but changing the rhythms. Make sure to practice these examples with a metronome to ensure accuracy, always at a slow, comfortable tempo. Don't worry—speed will come naturally in time. The most important thing is not to compromise your tone by trying to play too fast.

Example 7

Example 8a

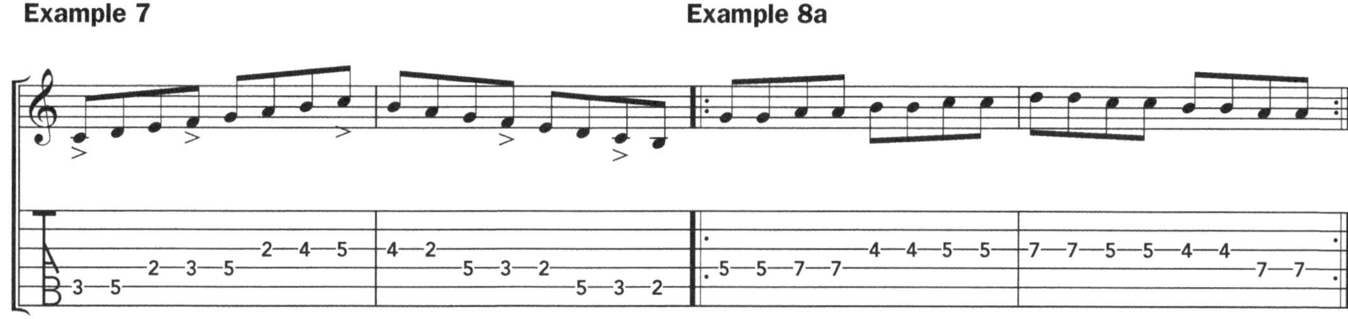

Example 8b

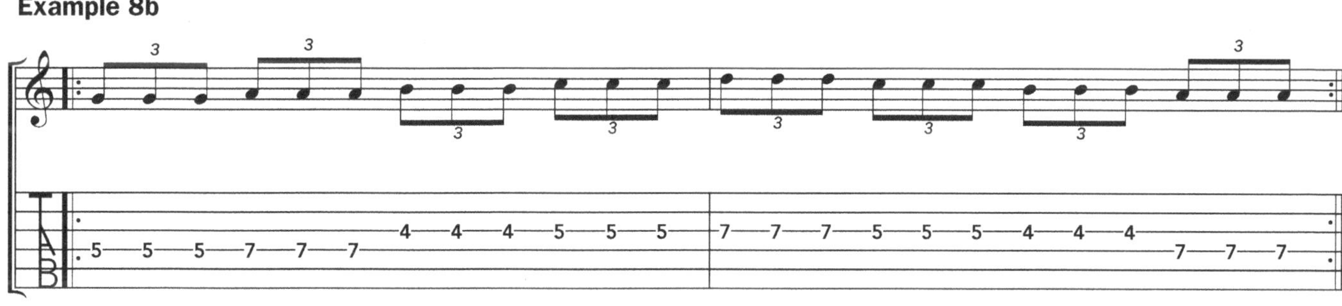

Example 8c

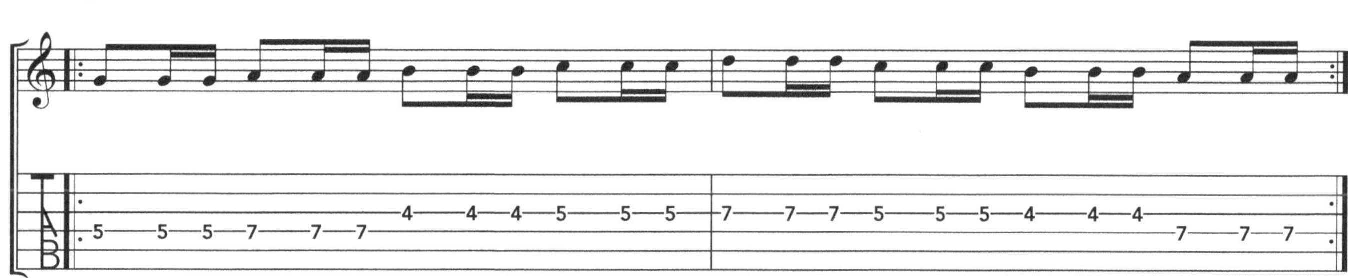

Example 8d

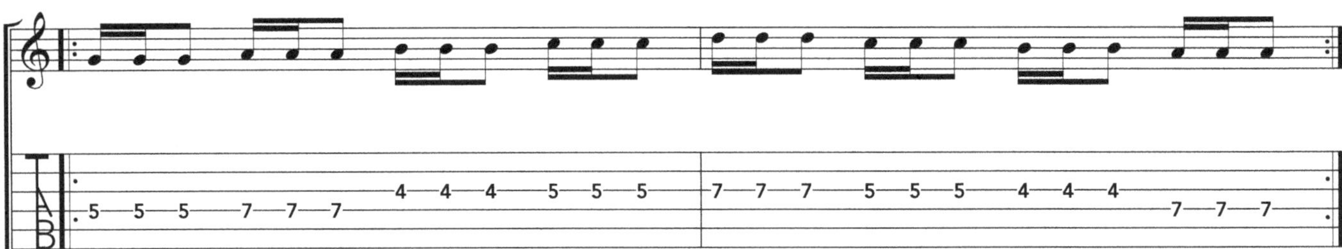

Example 8e

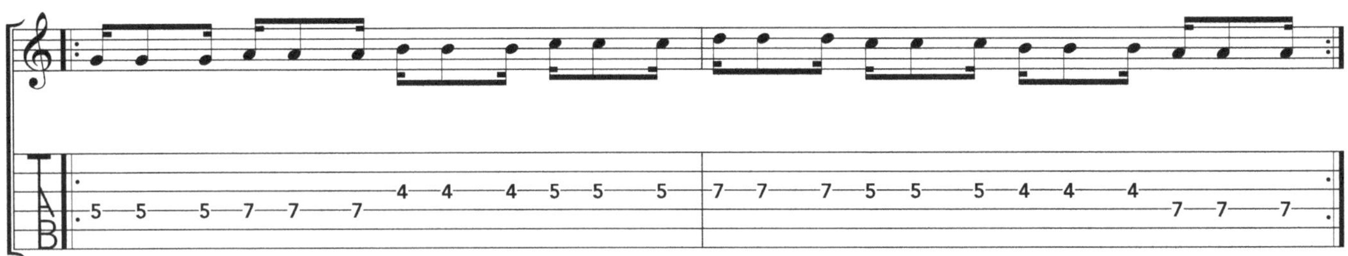

Example 8f

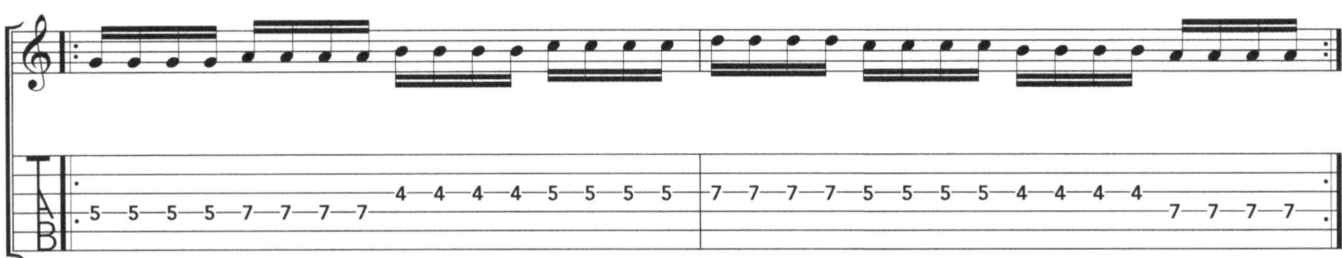

Example 9

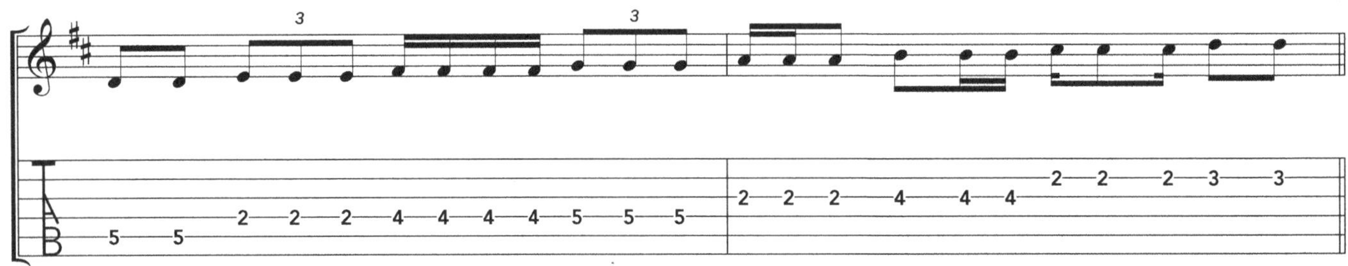

Example 10

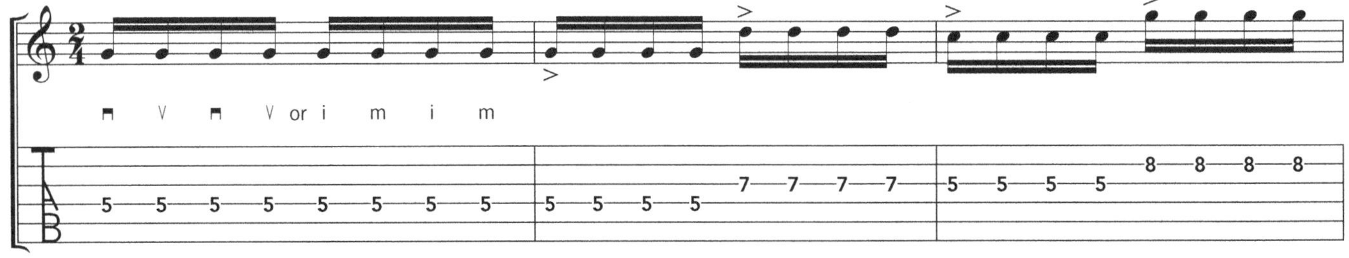

After you've practiced these, try playing **Example 9**, which moves through a D major scale (D E F# G A B C#) mixing all the rhythms. Imagine you are a drummer playing these rhythms on a snare, alternating between the left and right hands (corresponding to up- and down-strokes). Work through the different rhythmic combinations, and really settle in to creating a strong time feel. In fact, we can use common drum rudiments to develop picking dexterity.

Examples 10–13 introduce the single-stroke roll, single-stroke four (using triplet rhythms), and the single and double paradiddles crossing string sets. Notice the accents in the musical notation, as these will bring the examples to life. You can also experiment with contrasts in volume as with the earlier examples.

Example 11

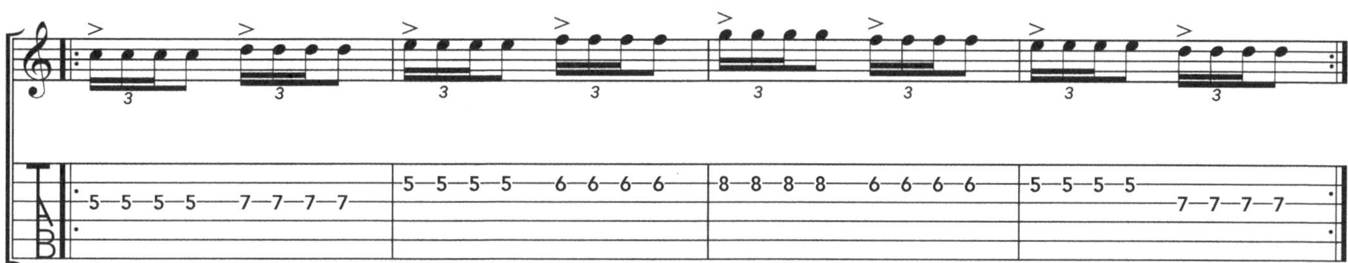

Example 12

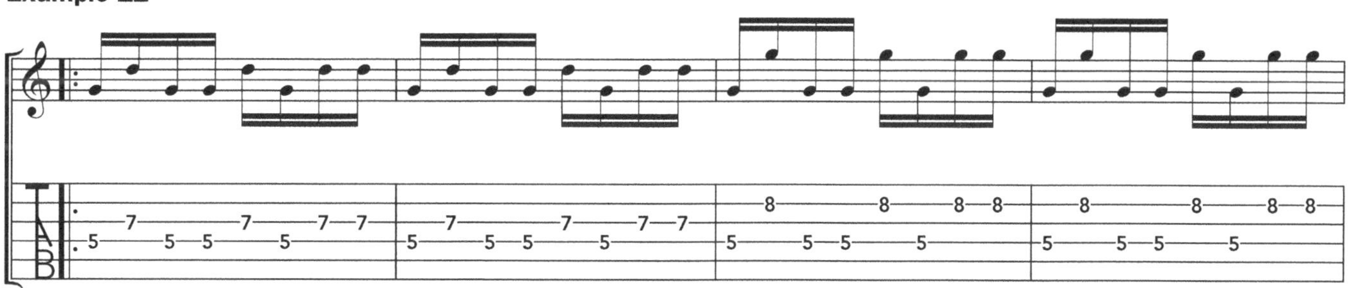

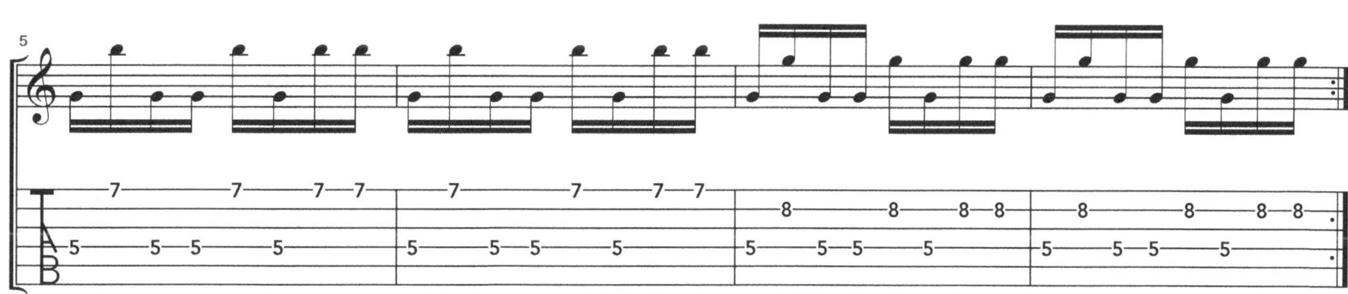

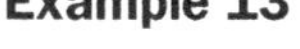

Example 13

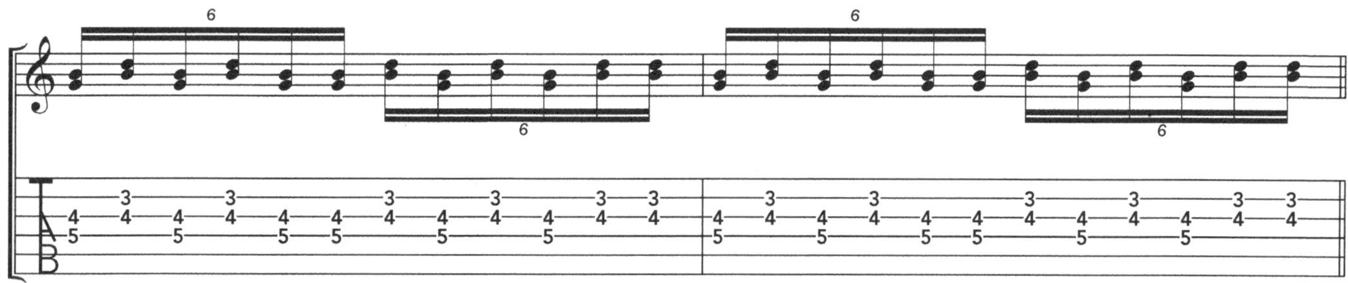

When considering articulation in the fretting hand, the most common techniques are hammer-ons, pull-offs, and slides (in time or quick, grace notes). **Example 14** shows a riff in C major where the notes on each string are connected using an ascending or descending slide. Pick each note and then use the fingers on the fretting hand to slide up or down, keeping the sound of the notes uninterrupted and full. In beats 3 and 4, pick the note once and then slide up and down with the fingers.

You can also slide between notes of larger intervals for a vocal-like phrasing effect. **Example 15a** slides an E up to a G; **Example 15b** starts all the way down on the C in the first position and slides up a fifth to the G. Try sliding with the finger that makes sense to play the remaining notes in the phrase. For instance, in both examples, try your third finger so you can use your first and second to finish out the phrase. If you use your first finger to slide, you won't be able to quickly and efficiently play the notes starting on the third beat.

Example 16 illustrates the use of sliding into grace notes from above or below. This technique is like a flam on a snare drum. You don't want to hear two different rhythms; rather, the grace note is played right on the beat and immediately slides up or down into the target note. These work best when played one fret above or below the target note. For a more dramatic effect, **Example 17** works through a C major scale with slides connecting every other note. Practicing these exercises will also sharpen your physical acuity in shifting positions around the fretboard.

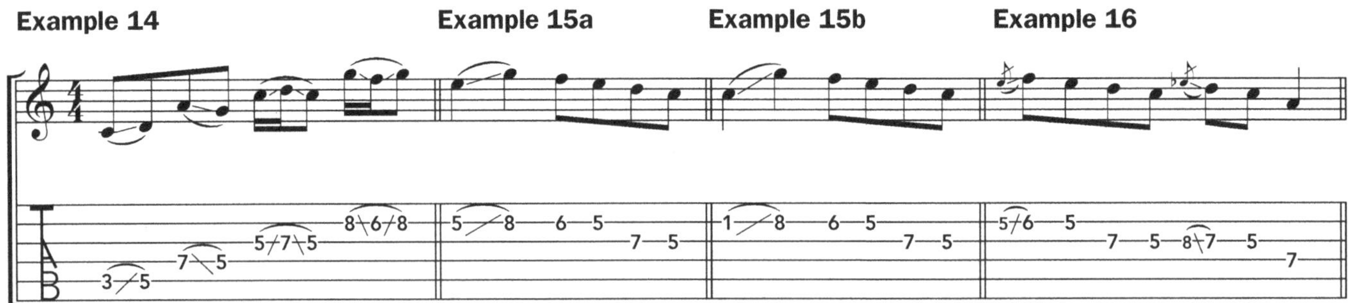

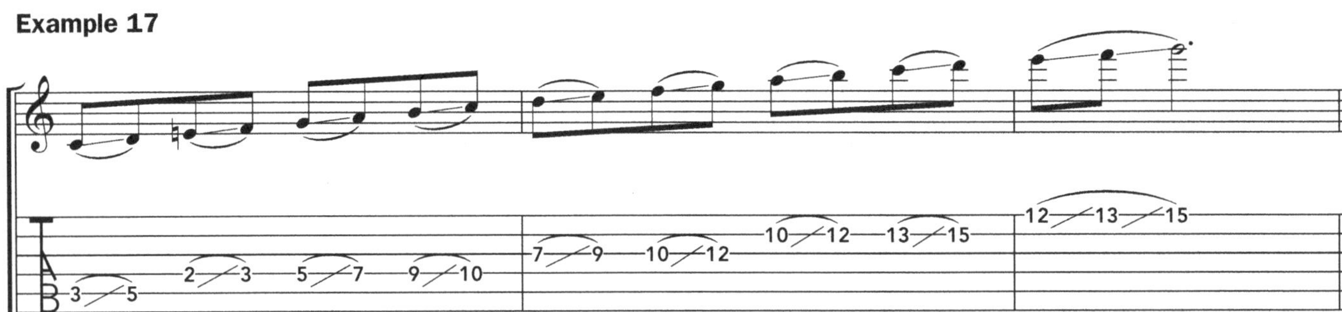

The most common articulation on the guitar, in addition to picking, is the use of hammer-ons and pull-offs, as shown in **Examples 18a–b**. When playing a hammer-on, pick the first note and then swing the second, third, or fourth finger onto the following note, making sure to connect squarely with the fretboard with the tip of the finger. Pull-offs generally start with the fourth, third, or second finger pulling the string down towards the floor—almost in a flicking motion—while the first finger is already in position fretting the following desired note.

You can use more than one hammer-on or pull-off in succession, as demonstrated in **Example 19**. Note the position shift on the G string; the notes A and B are hammered using the first and third fingers. Following a quick shift to fifth position, the first and third fingers hammer the C onto the D note. In the third measure, repeat the following with the third finger pulling off to the first finger in both positions.

Developing facility and endurance with these techniques is important to all styles of guitar playing, and playing hammer-on/pull-off combinations between two notes on a string is excellent to practice. **Examples 20–21** demonstrate this using major and Kumoi pentatonic scales with two notes per string.

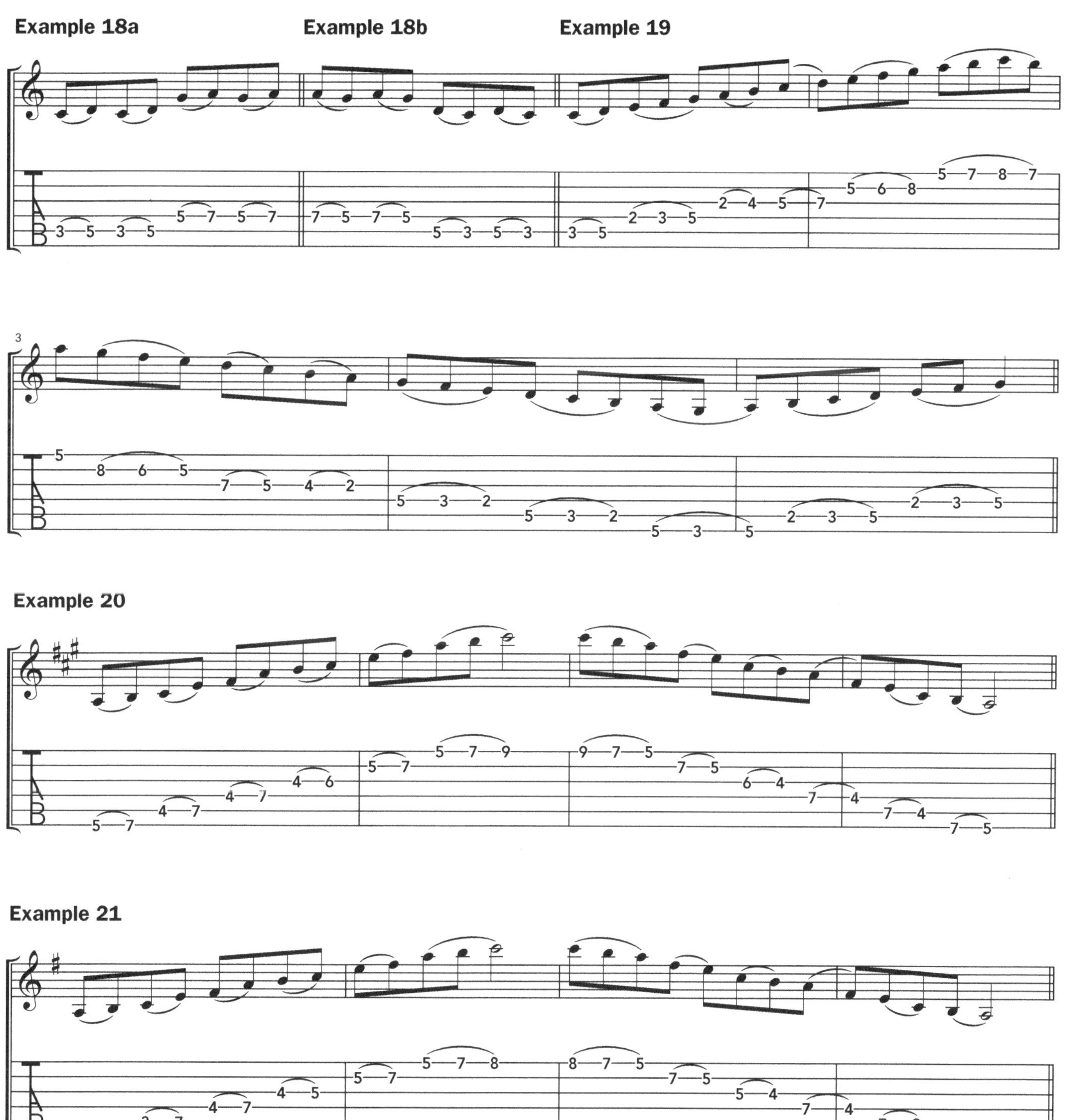

Example 22 expands on this by adding a double hammer-on/pull-off on each string, while **Example 23** crosses up and down the various strings.

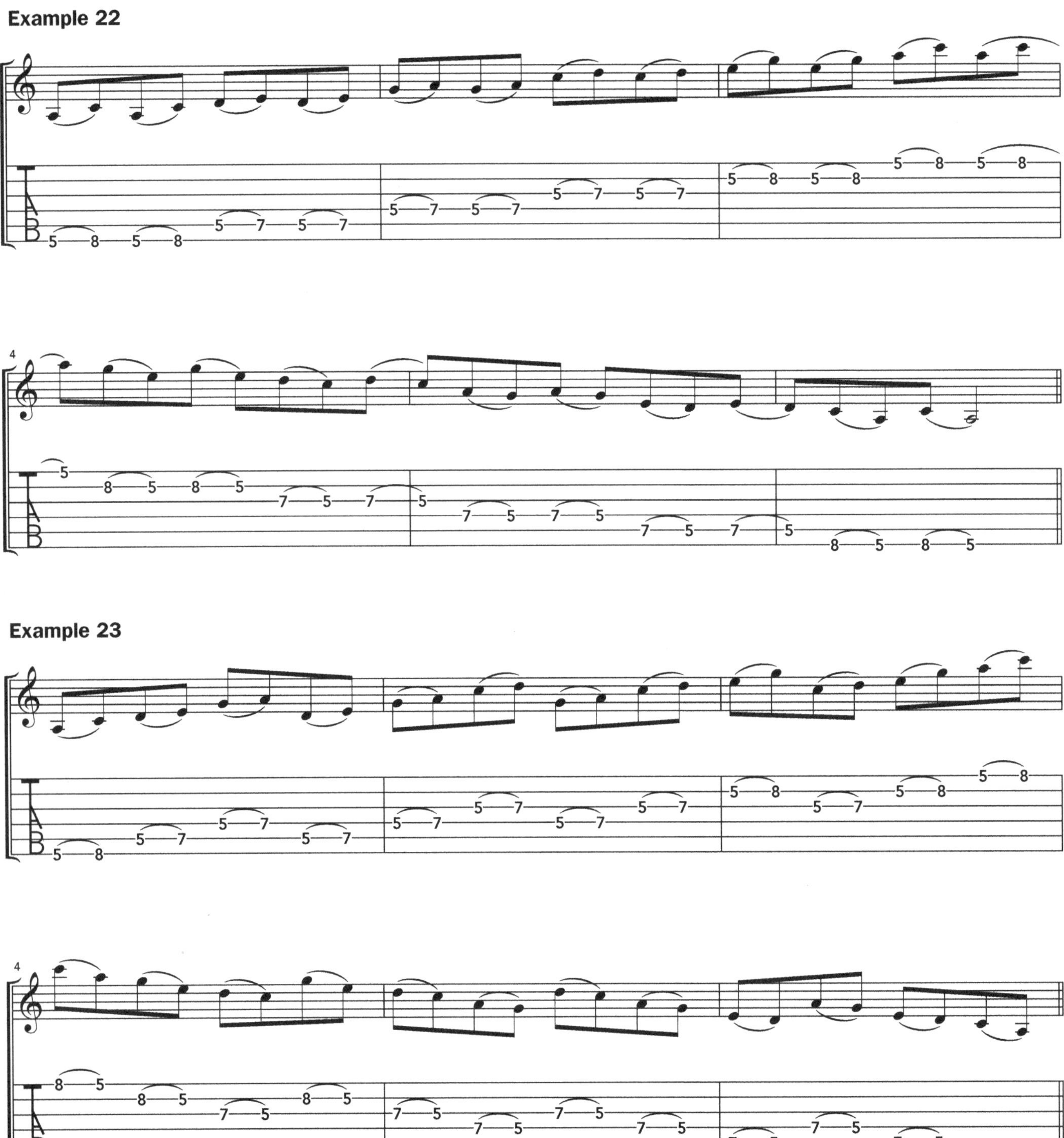

Example 24 is a short étude that focuses on using hammer-ons and pull-offs with major and minor triad shapes. These exercises are great but can also be strenuous. Be careful not to play these too hard or long, and make sure to take a break as soon as you feel any type of pain or cramping in your fretting hand. Slowly but surely, you will develop a considerable amount of endurance by practicing these examples. And remember to always strive for a full, clear sound.

Example 24

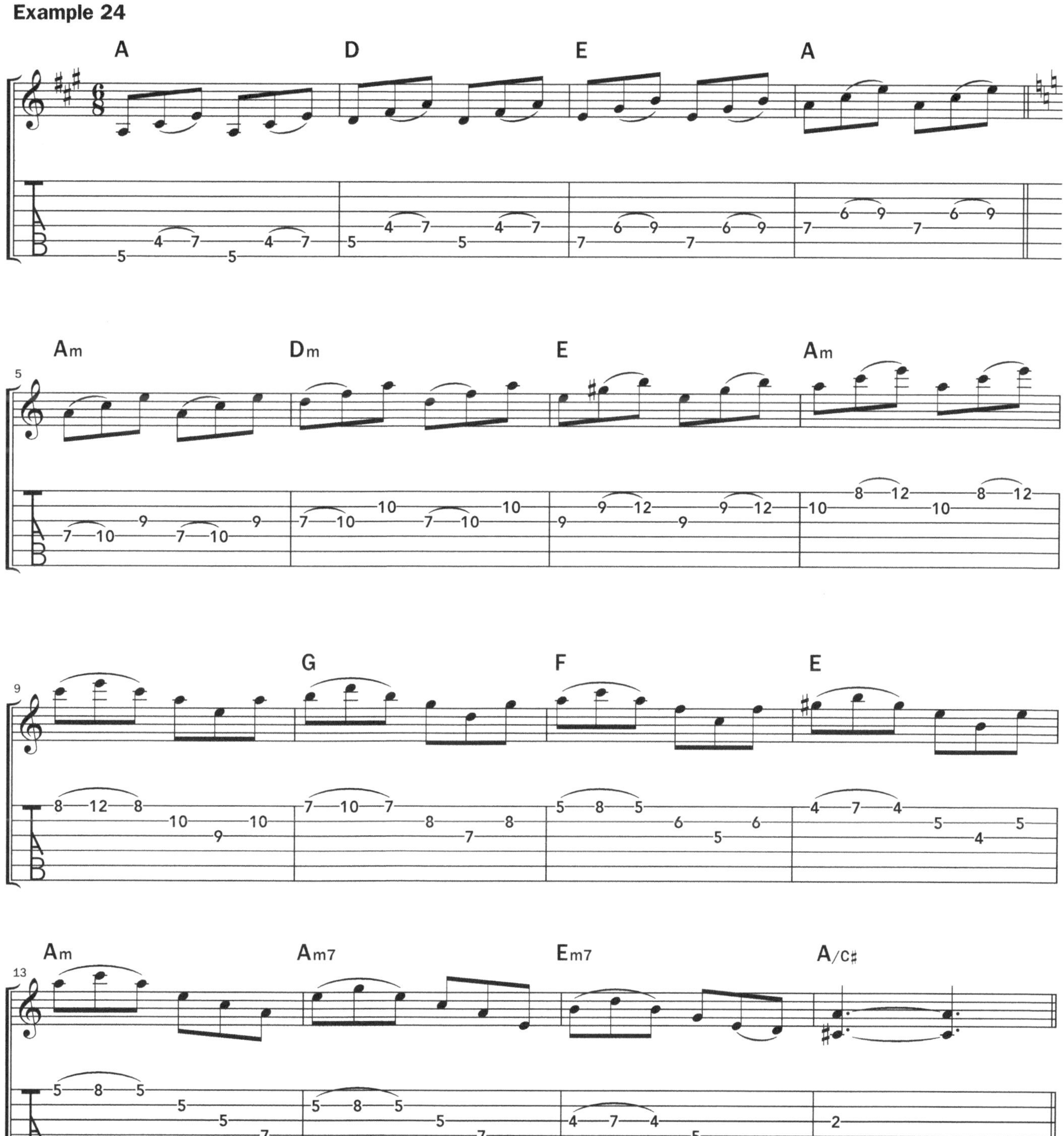

Refining Technique: Coordination and Control

Now let's home in on developing control between the fingers of the fretting hand, and between the fretting and picking hands. **Example 25** is a wonderful exercise that develops coordination using pairs of finger combinations working through a chromatic scale in octaves. Pay close attention to the fingering indicated in the TAB as you will be alternating mostly between the first and third and the second and fourth fingers. While it may seem frustrating at first, stick with it and play it very slowly. This will ultimately pay dividends with regard to finger control and independence in all styles of playing.

Developing technique doesn't necessarily mean playing scales and arpeggios. **Example 26** is an exercise that emphasizes the difference between long (legato) and short (staccato) notes within a chord. The Cmaj7 chord in the example has four notes, each played by a separate finger. Imagine each note or finger is a voice. Now imagine one of the notes is held long while the other three are staccato (as short as possible).

The first bar has the top note E held by the fourth finger. While that digit frets the note and stays held down, the other three fingers quickly release pressure from the strings. They don't even need to leave the strings; just release the pressure while the pinky stays down, holding the sustained note. In the next measure, the B is sustained by the second finger. Now the first, third, and fourth fingers will all bounce back, as if they were touching a hot stove. Continue this through the following measures as the sustained notes and chord voicings change.

Example 27 depicts a challenging exercise playing through three different chord arpeggios in tenths. Experiment with different fretting hand fingerings—always trying to plot out fingerings in advance to ensure smooth continuity—and use either hybrid picking or fingerstyle techniques with the other hand. **Examples 28–29** work on string crossing, one of the most challenging synchronization techniques to master on guitar, with different types of triads, and then diatonic seventh chords in the key of D major ascending through string sets and fretboard positions.

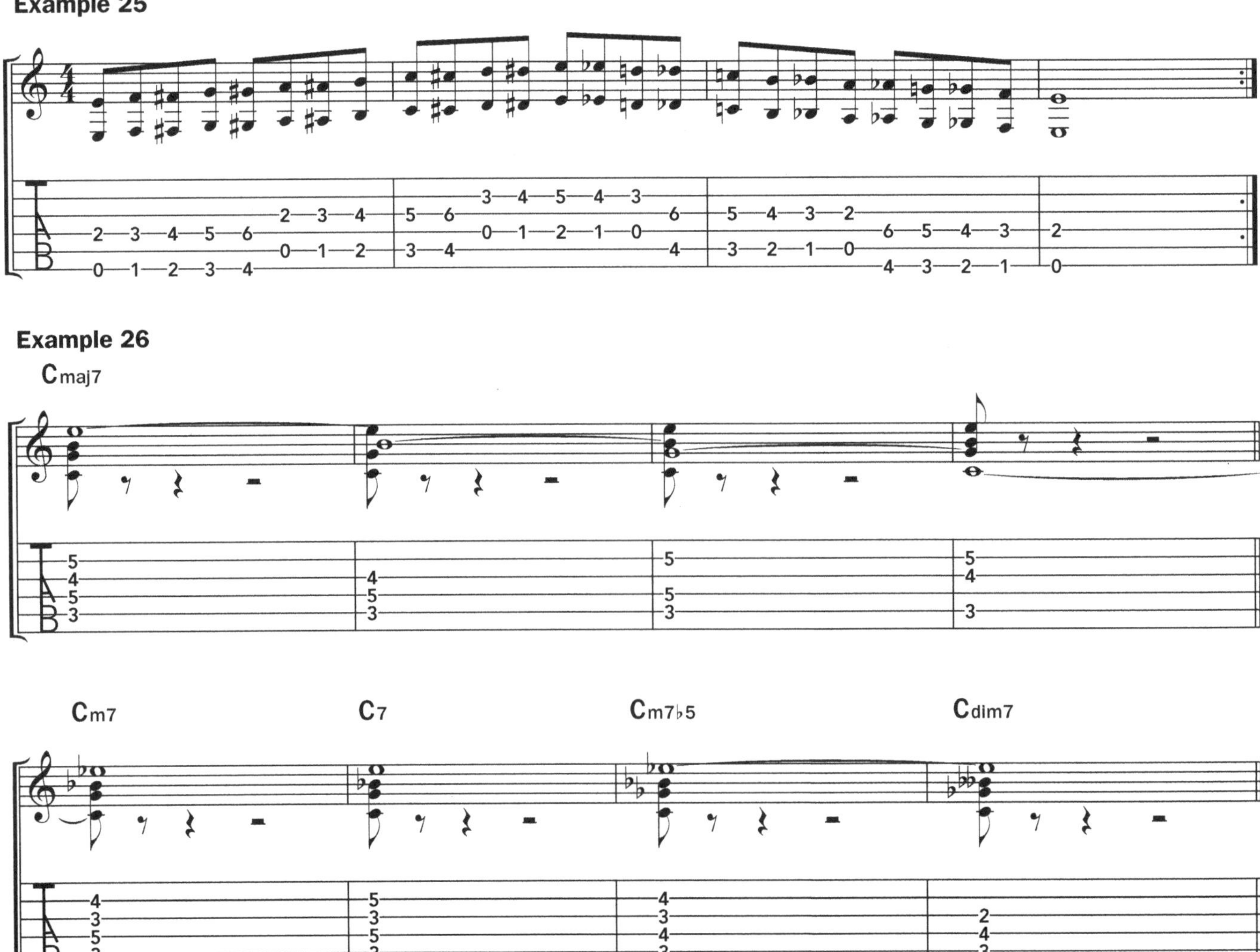

Example 27

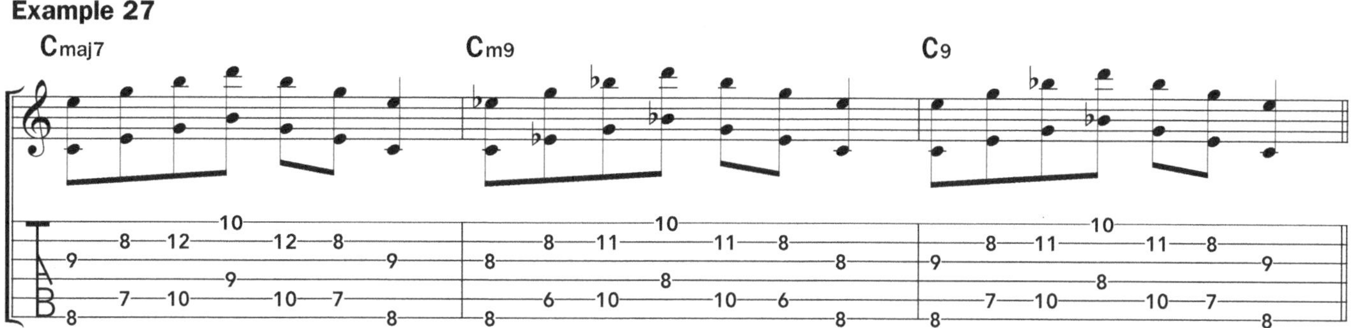

Example 28

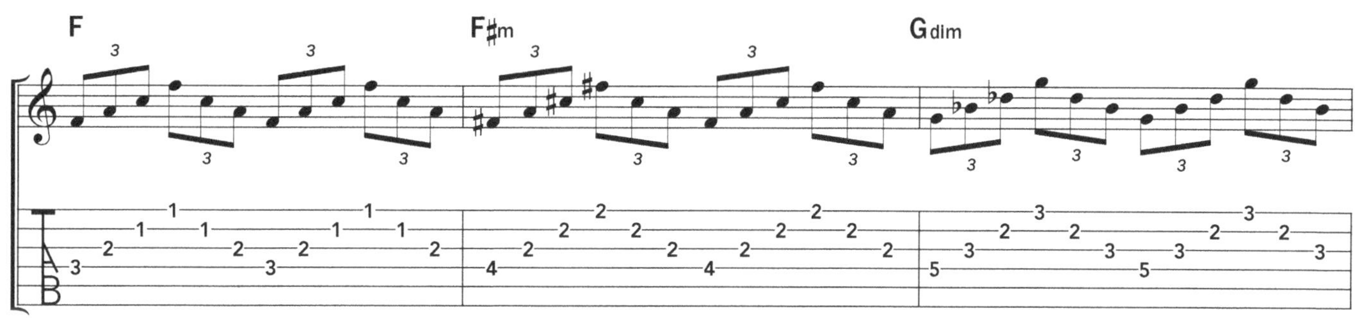

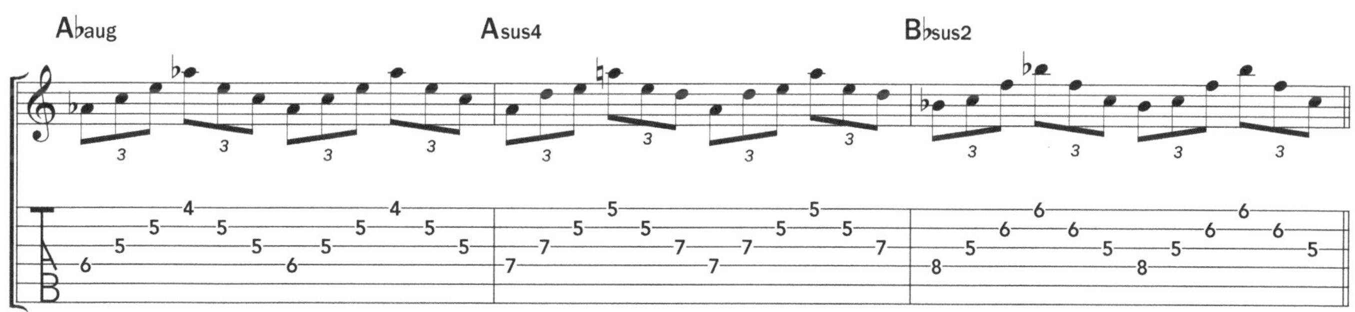

Example 29

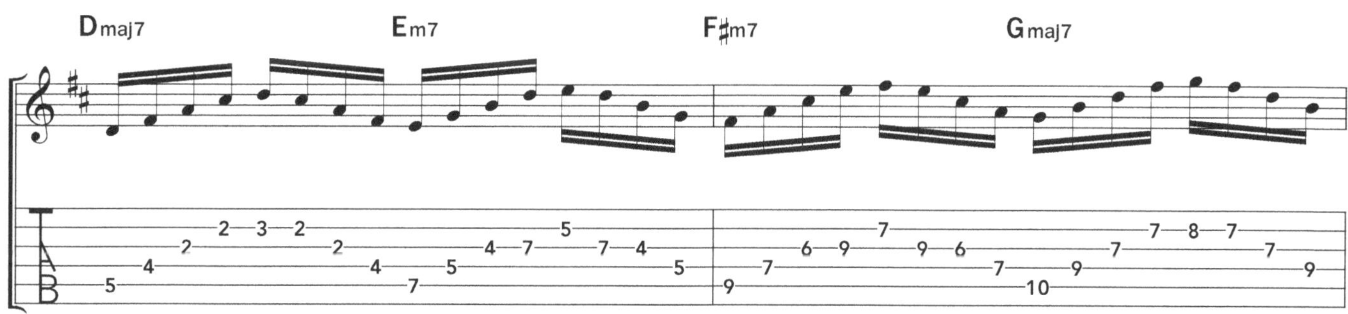

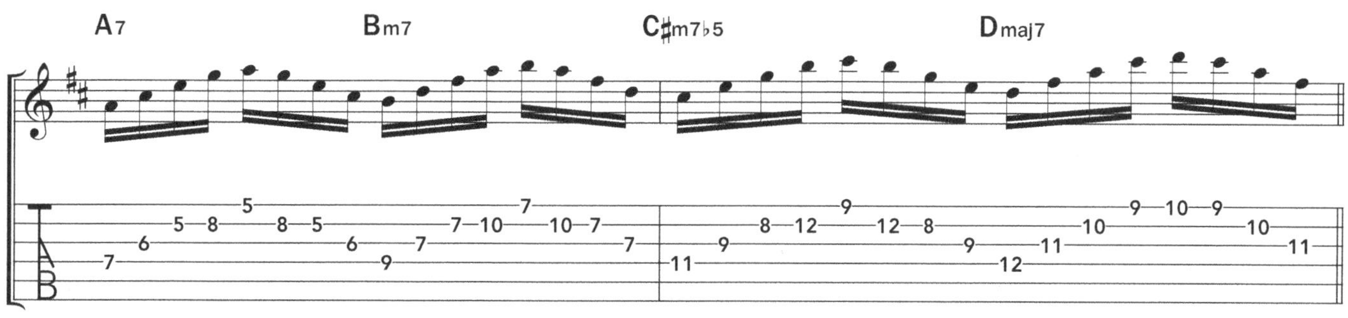

Taking coordination to the next level, **Examples 30–31** incorporate string skipping with crossing using diatonic triads and scale combinations in D major. Try writing out your own variations on these concepts with different chords and harmonies, for instance, ascending through an arpeggio and descending with a scale, or vice versa.

The next few examples work through sweep (also known as "directional" or "economy") picking. The concept is to finger an arpeggio in the fretting hand using one note per string, while the pick uses consecutive down- or up-strokes. The result can be astonishingly rapid flurries of notes to create different textures in solos. To achieve this effect playing fingerstyle, you can either sweep using the thumb (p) or a rapid combination of thumb, index, middle, and/or ring fingers (p-i-m-a).

Example 30

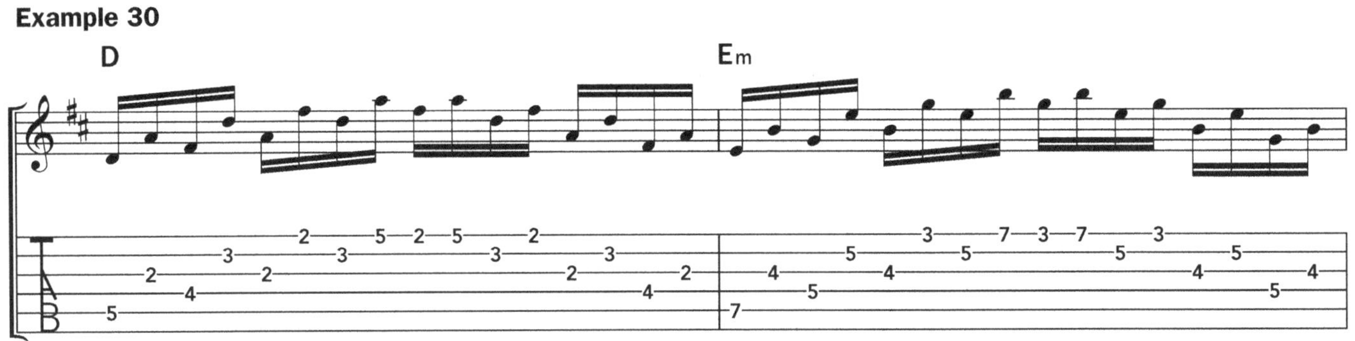

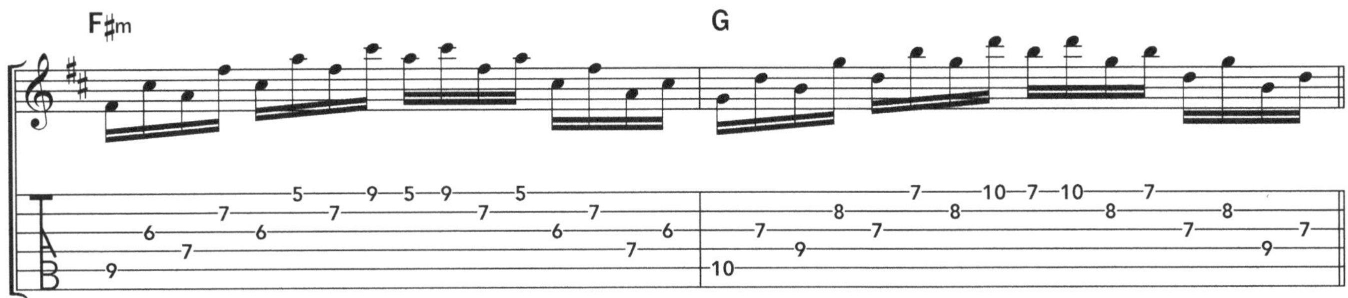

Example 31

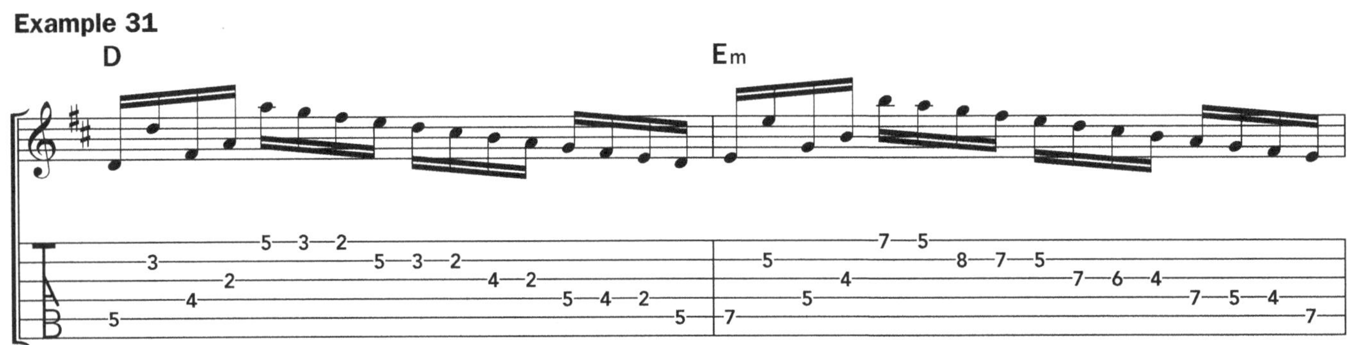

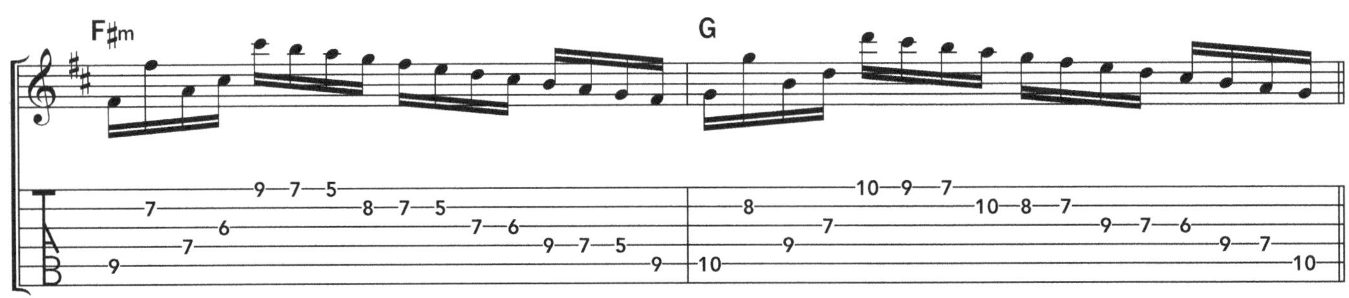

Example 32 illustrates the basic premise of the technique. Working through diatonic triads on three or four strings is a great way to get acclimated to this technique, either using a pick or fingers. The idea is to create a flourish of notes that is distinct from alternate picking but still has inherently solid rhythm. The fretting hand will maintain the shape of the chord, but you can experiment with a rolling technique of the fingers releasing pressure after the notes have been articulated, keeping the final note in the passage held down, as in the example.

Example 33 takes this concept a step further by following each arpeggio with a descending scale pattern. For this example, sweep the first four notes of each arpeggio and follow by using alternate picking for the descending scale, as indicated in the music notation. **Example 34** illustrates the same concept in reverse—using an upstroke sweep—with a common rhythmic pattern used in modern jazz, rock, and bluegrass solos.

Example 32

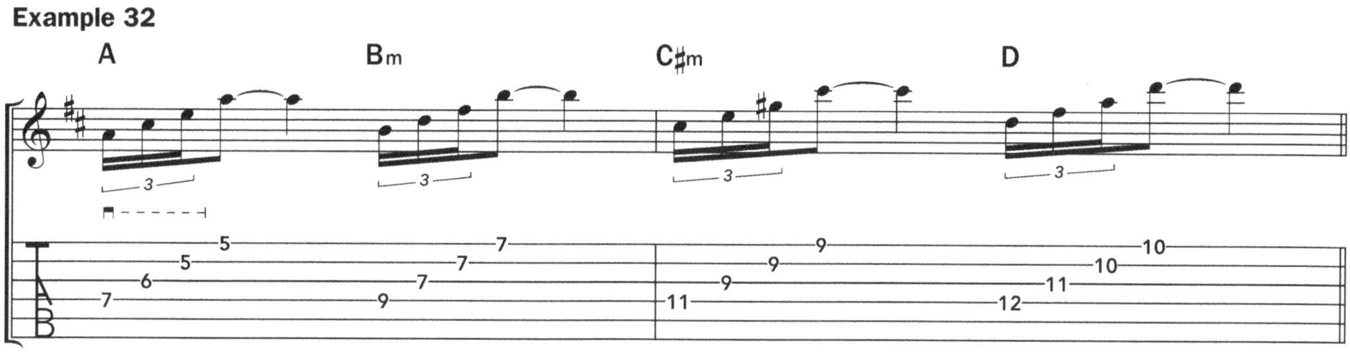

Example 33

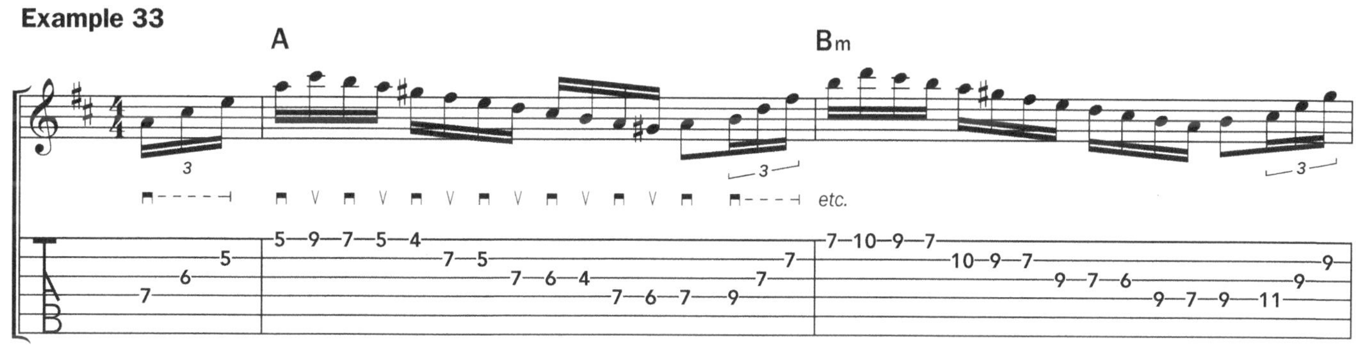

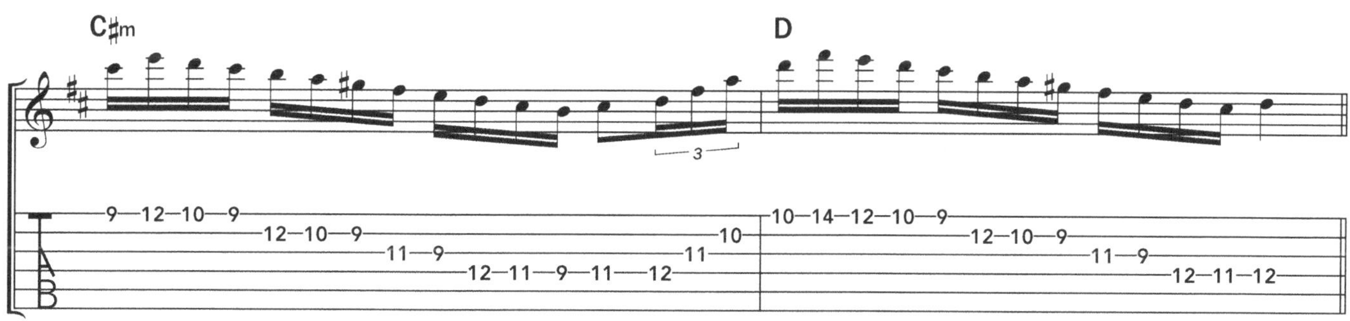

Example 34

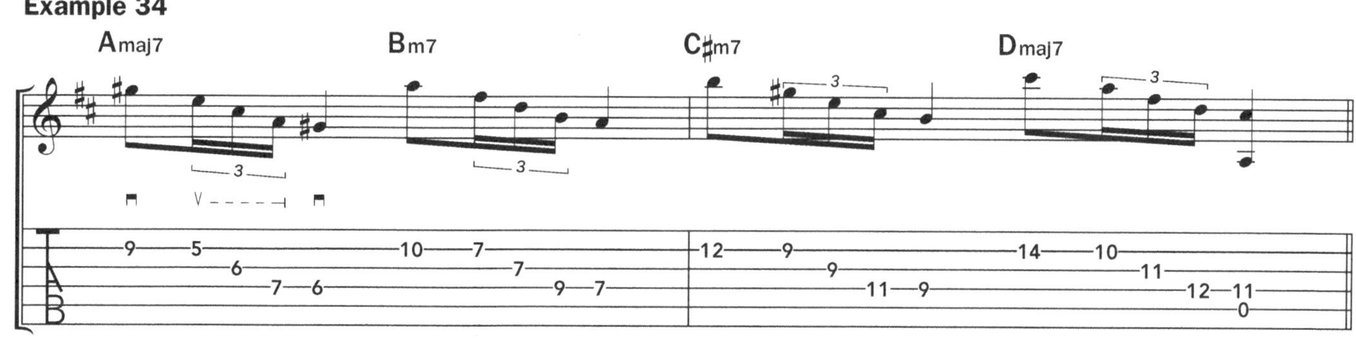

Putting It All Together

The ultimate goal, of course, is to develop enough technical proficiency to meet the demands of the music you love to play, all while expressing your own unique identity on the guitar. In addition to the exercises you've already worked through, it's important to play real music in every practice session so you can explore implementing these techniques and textures into your own repertoire.

The following excerpts, études, and pieces will present unique technical challenges in different styles, but keep in mind the concepts we've already practiced and developed, specifically: tone quality, dynamic expression, accenting, rhythmic precision, phrasing and articulation, and effortless control.

Example 35 is a common and well-loved traditional Irish jig called "Out in the Ocean," while **Example 36** is inspired by bebop pioneer Charlie Parker's improvised solo on "Anthropology." Trad/fiddle and jazz/bebop tunes can offer incredible opportunities to develop different techniques and chops, mainly because those intricate melodies weren't written for guitar. But if you can develop the ability to solve fingering and picking problems—and learn to phrase in a more legato manner, like a violin or saxophone—your guitar technique will improve by leaps and bounds.

The next two études were specifically composed to develop facility with arpeggios and scales. Matteo Carcassi's "Estudio No. 3" (from his time-honored collection *25 Estudios for Guitar, op. 60*) in **Example 37** provides a fantastic workout with chordal arpeggios for the picking hand, whether playing fingerstyle or with a flatpick.

"Invention No. 4" (**Example 38**) was composed by J.S. Bach as a keyboard étude, featuring two parts in counterpoint for each hand, exploring melodies, scales, and arpeggios in the key of D minor. Both parts are included here; try recording one part and playing along, or practicing with another guitarist to experience the incredible melodic and counterpoint sensibilities of Bach, as well as the inherent technical challenges.

Example 39 features an arrangement of Bach's beloved "Prelude in G Major, Cello Suite No. 1" from his *Six Cello Suites* masterpiece. This arrangement captures the extended range of a cello by using an alternate tuning: C G D G B E, low to high. This piece is equally challenging and rewarding when played fingerstyle or with a pick. Try to experiment with the melodic and rhythmic flow of the piece (listen to various recordings by cellists and classical guitarists) and allow the sonorous melodic strands to ring out in your phrasing and dynamics.

Example 35: "Out in the Ocean"

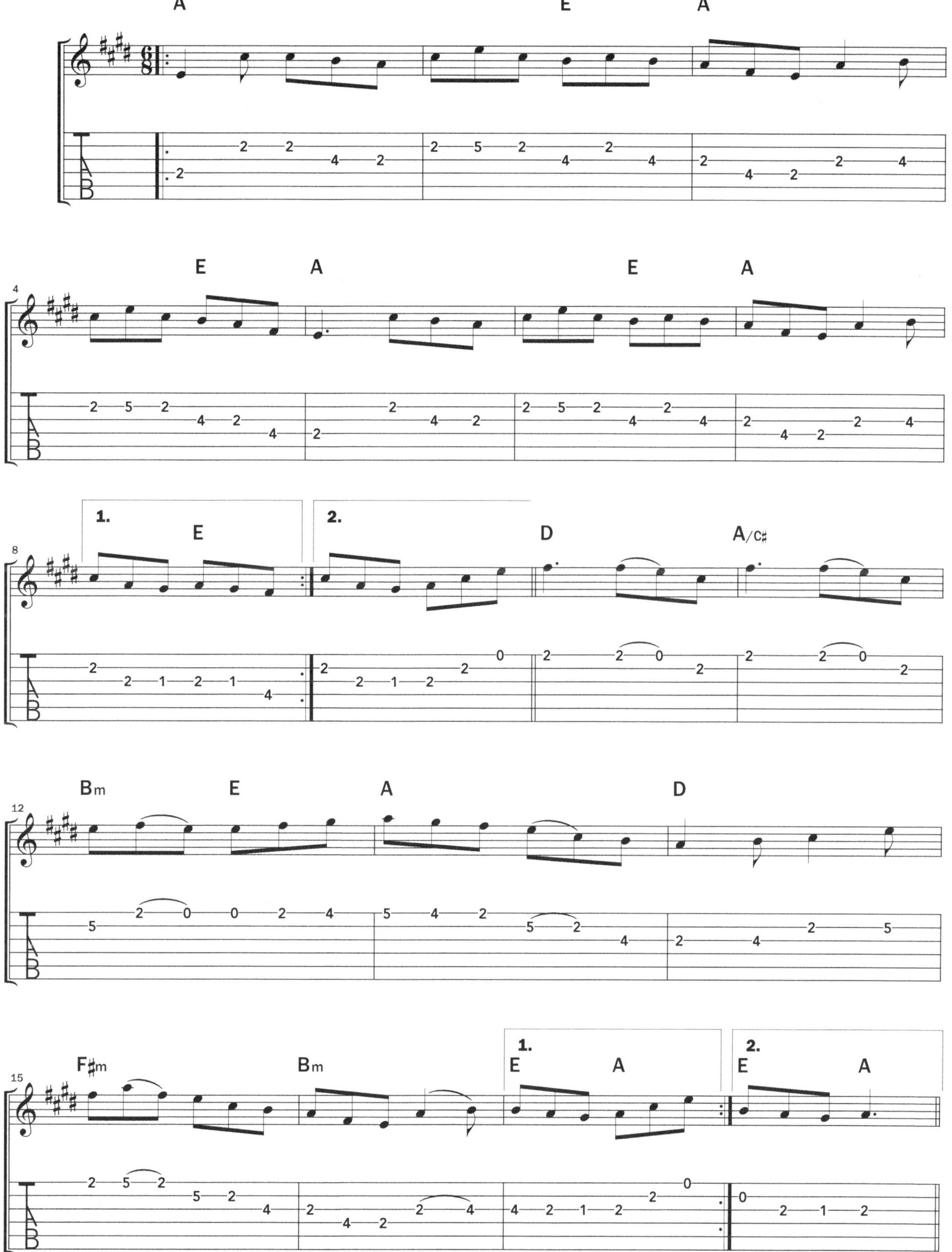

Example 36: à la "Anthropology"

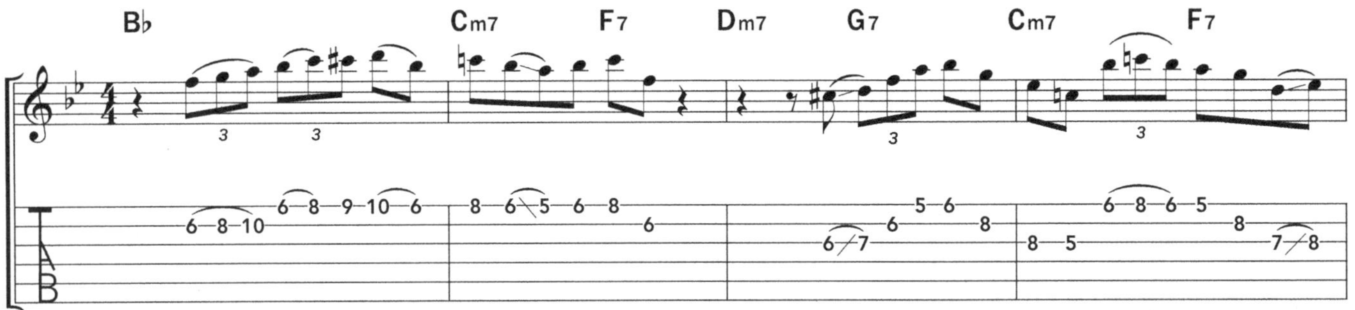

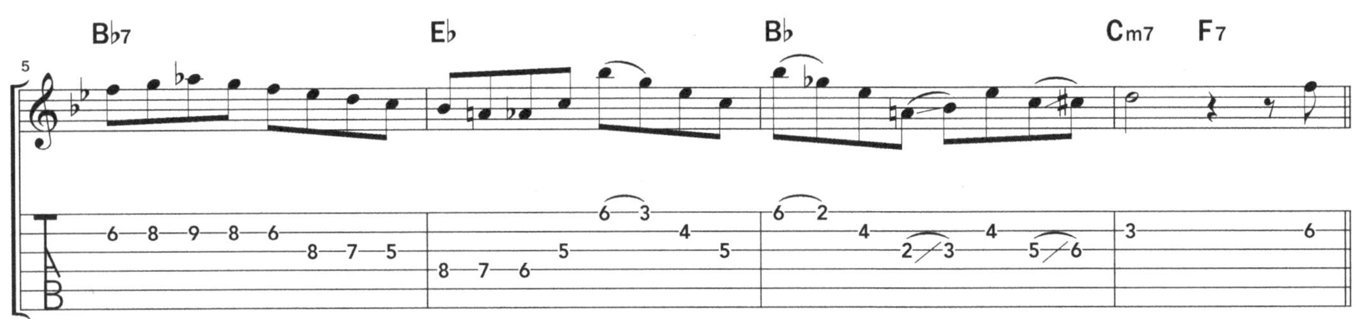

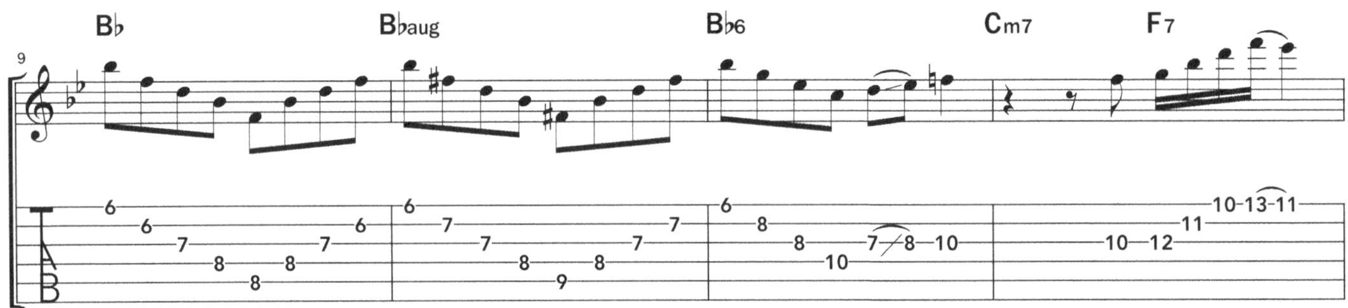

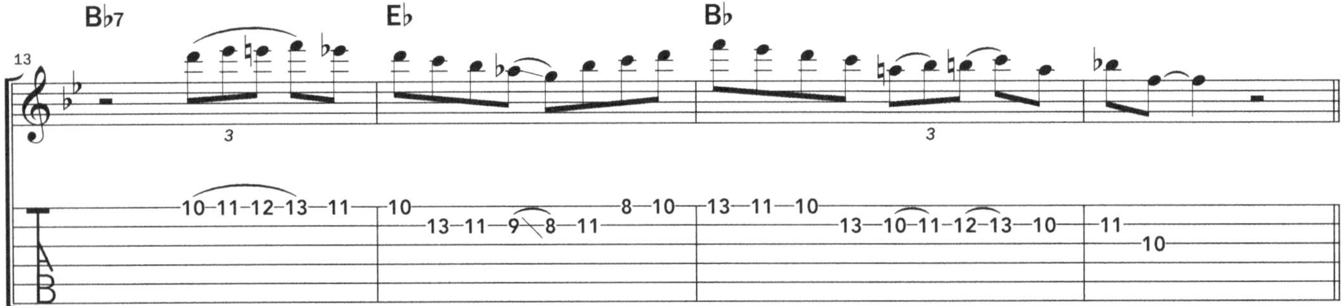

Learning to Read Music

Guitarists who are just learning to read music sometimes make the mistake of trying to read through a piece in its entirety, capturing all the pitches, rhythms, articulations, interpretations, etc., all of which are typically beyond their ability. The inevitable result? Frustration and a general dislike of sight-reading.

Instead, learning to read should be broken down into different elements: pitch recognition, knowledge of rhythm, accessing the notes on the fretboard, and interpretation (including stylistic, chord symbols, and dynamics). By separating each of these elements and practicing them individually, your reading abilities will markedly improve in a relatively short time.

To work on pitch recognition, fill out a blank piece of staff paper with random black dots. Don't use any rhythms or accidentals (sharps or flats) to start with, just plain black dots on a line or space. Find a tempo on your metronome that is relatively slow but also provides just a little challenge (increasing the tempo as you start to improve and/or memorize the notes). Recite the note names out loud in time with the metronome and try to look ahead as much as you can—especially as you reach the end of a line. Once you've done this, repeat from the top of the page, but this time, recite the notes out loud and play them, perhaps in a CAGED position you are familiar with.

Finally, go through the same exercise just playing the notes while thinking of the names silently in your mind. The most important thing to practice throughout this exercise is to not drop the time and lose your place on the page. If you're looking ahead and you know you can't name or play the note, just skip it and go to the next note. But whatever you do, don't drop the time or lose your place. In this way, you're not only practicing naming pitches on a staff, but you're practicing the art of staying in time and keeping your place in the music. This practice should be applied to rhythm reading as well.

In the same way you've isolated pitches and note placement on the fretboard, it's important to isolate rhythmic phrases. I recommend getting a book of snare drum études or material that illustrates various rhythms exclusively. Make sure to work out of a book that explores eighth-note, 16th-note, and triplet rhythms and subdivisions, as well as various time signatures and cut time feels.

Reading rhythms is just like reading language. Initially, you put letters together to form sounds and then words, which then form to create short phrases. Those phrases become complete sentences that transform into cohesive paragraphs to express ideas and information. Rhythm is the same. At first, you want to subdivide and count out the rhythms on each beat, and gradually you will recognize a rhythm over the course of two to four beats, and finally several measures. You'll be able to look at an entire rhythmic phrase and hear it in your head.

Interpretation will come with experience in various styles, learning to play at different dynamic levels and articulating crescendos and decrescendos. This should be a part of your technique practice. Think of a volume knob that has six settings and visualize what each would sound like. Now apply the same visualization to your hands. How hard do you need to strike the string to establish mezzo forte? Then, play softer or louder from there once you've established a dynamic ground zero.

Quite often guitar music will be in the form of a chord chart, so it's important to know solid workhorse voicings that will work in different styles. For instance, a G major chord voicing will be different in bluegrass, rock, pop, country, and jazz settings. By listening to a lot of different styles and studying the voicings and rhythmic language, you'll be much better positioned to come up with creative and stylistically appropriate guitar parts over otherwise nebulous charts.

Example 37: "Estudio No. 3 Andantino" by Matteo Carcassi

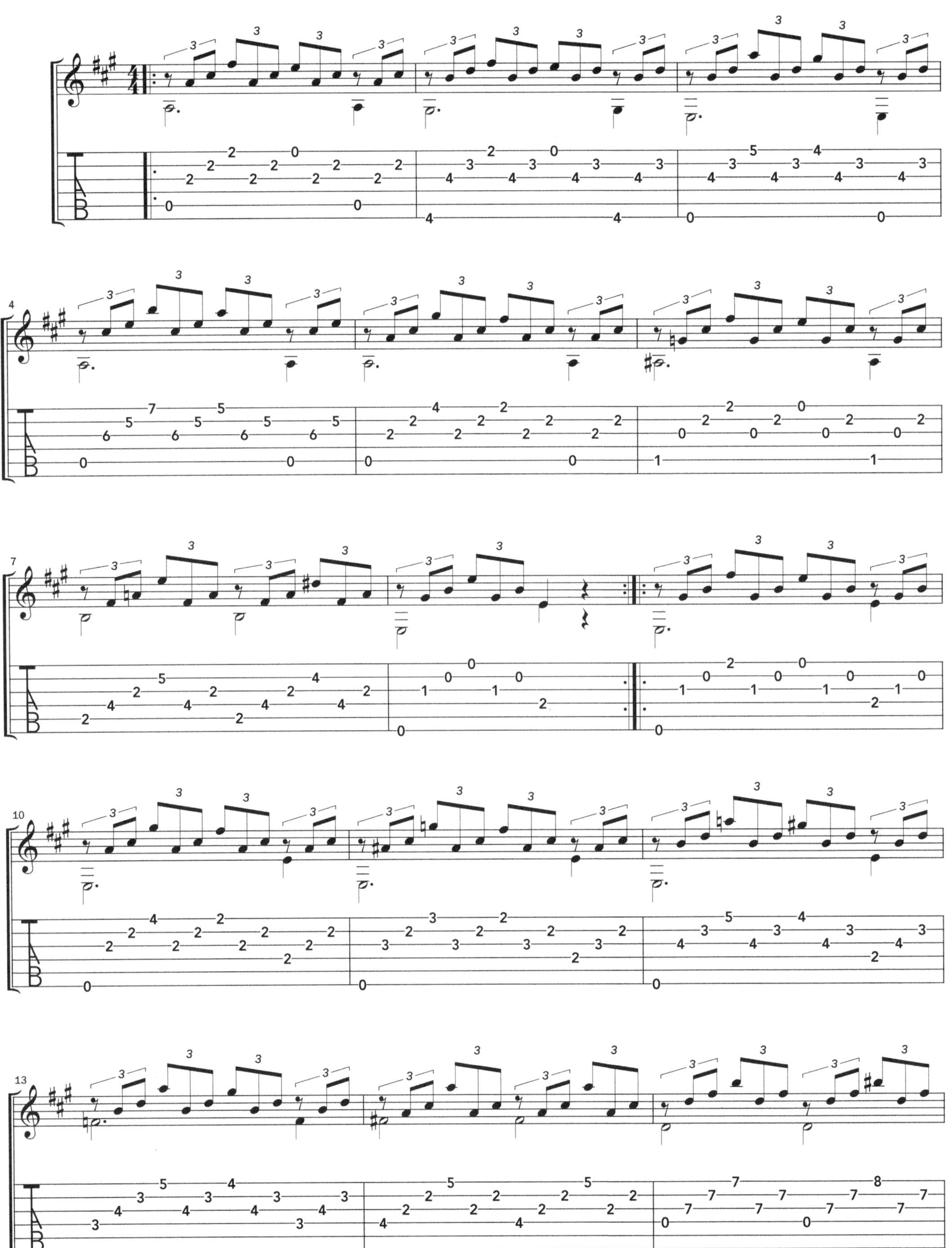

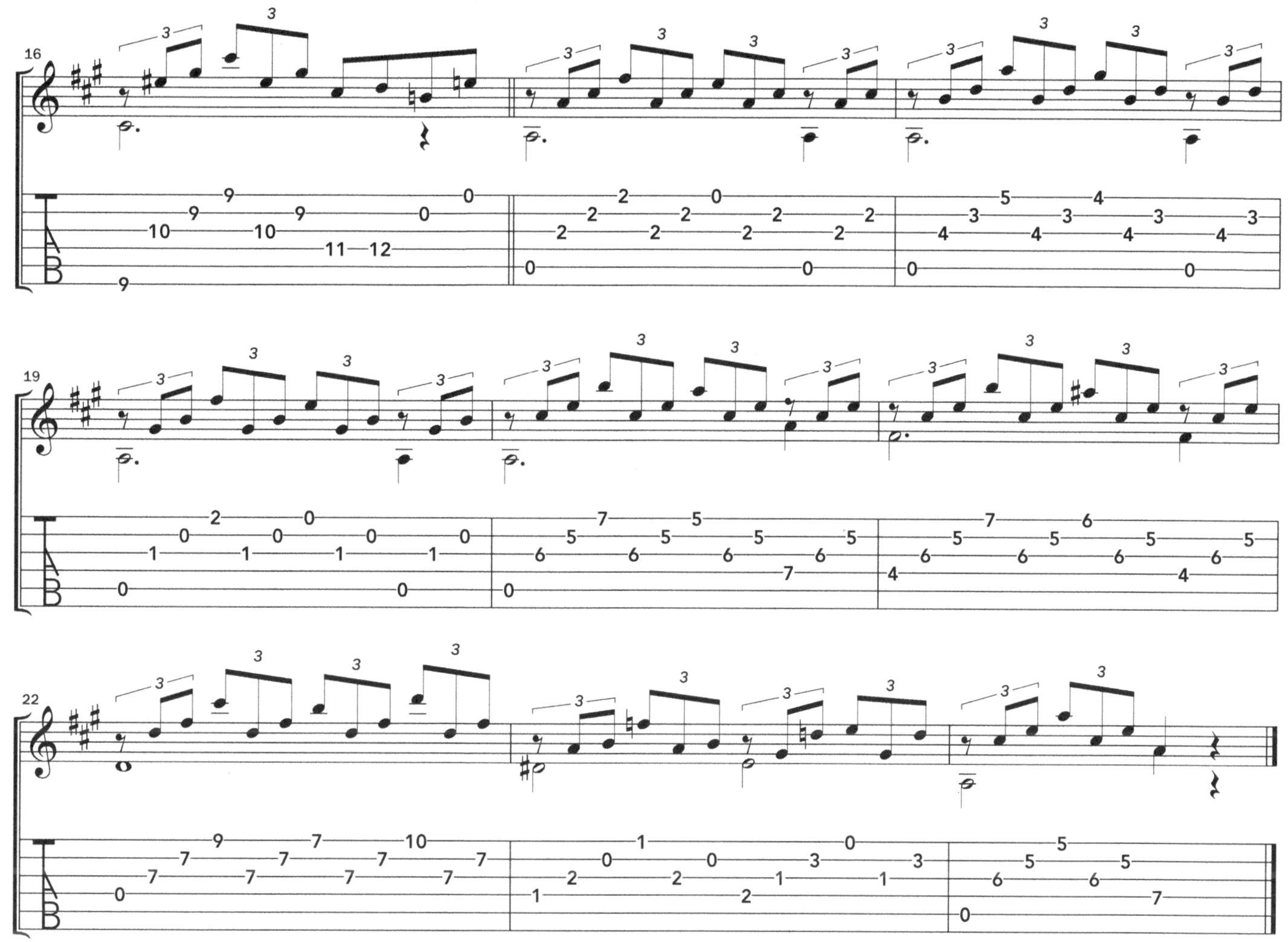

Example 38: "Invention No. 4" by J.S. Bach

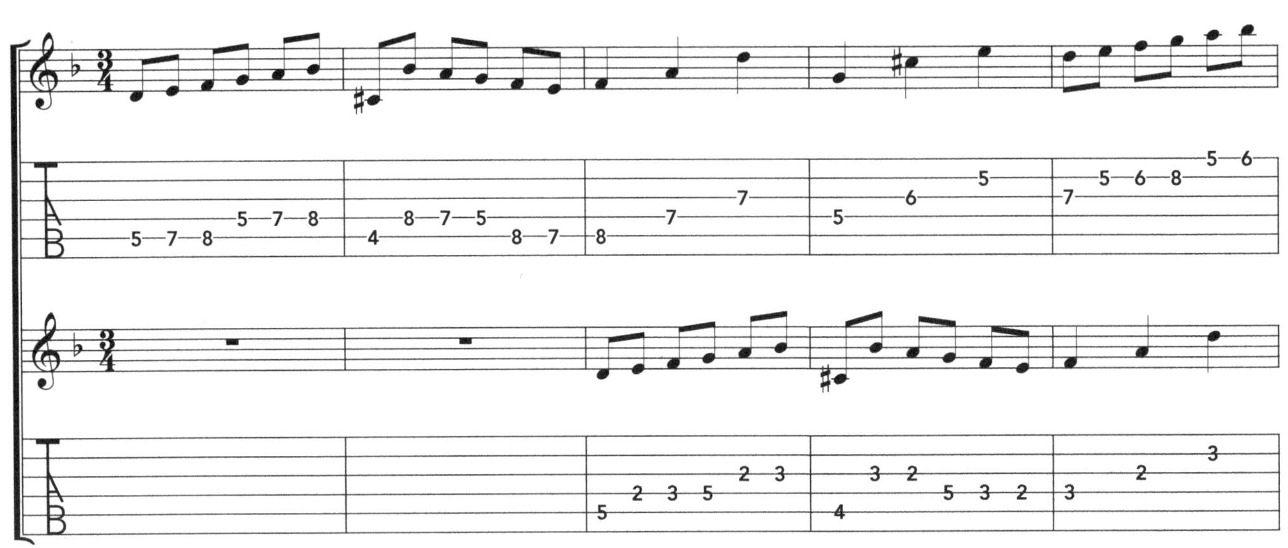

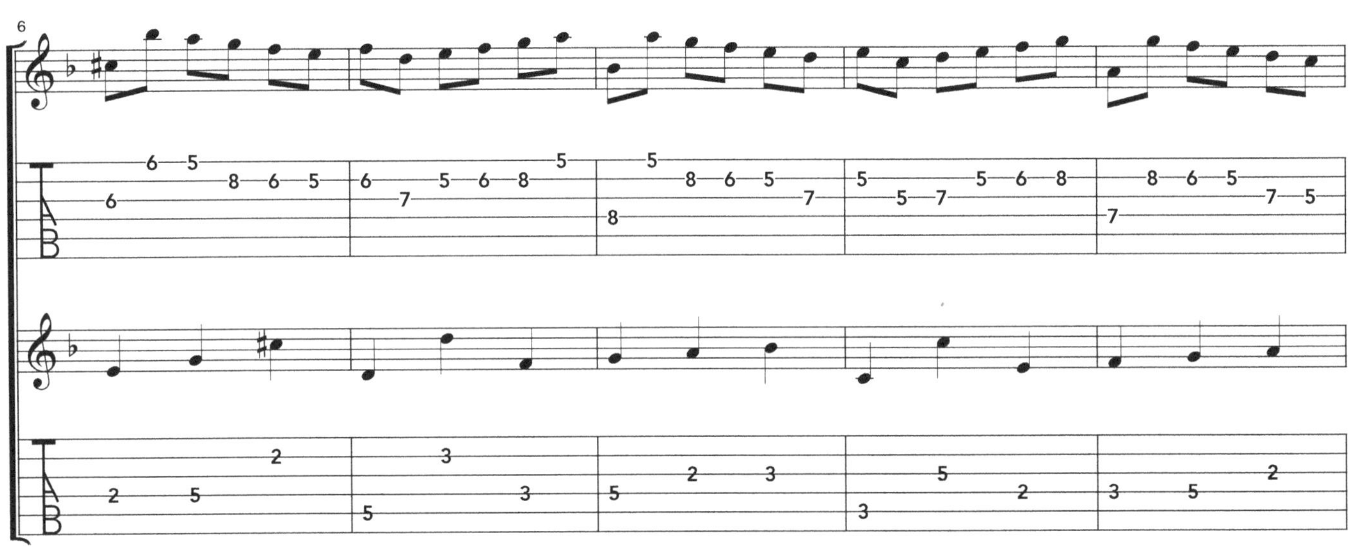

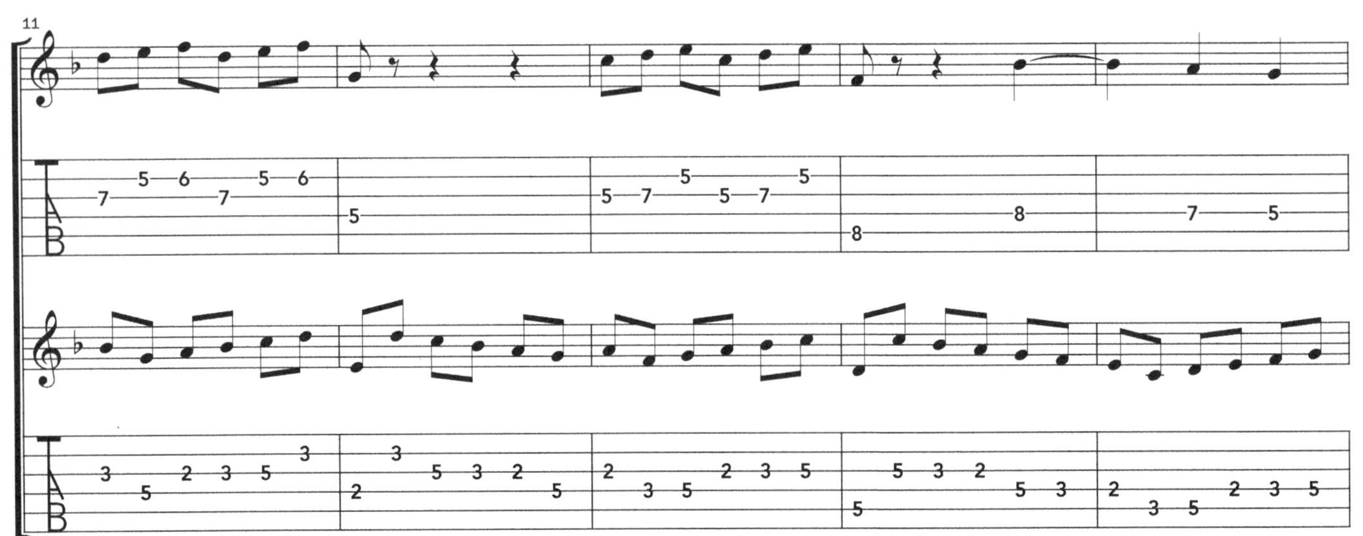

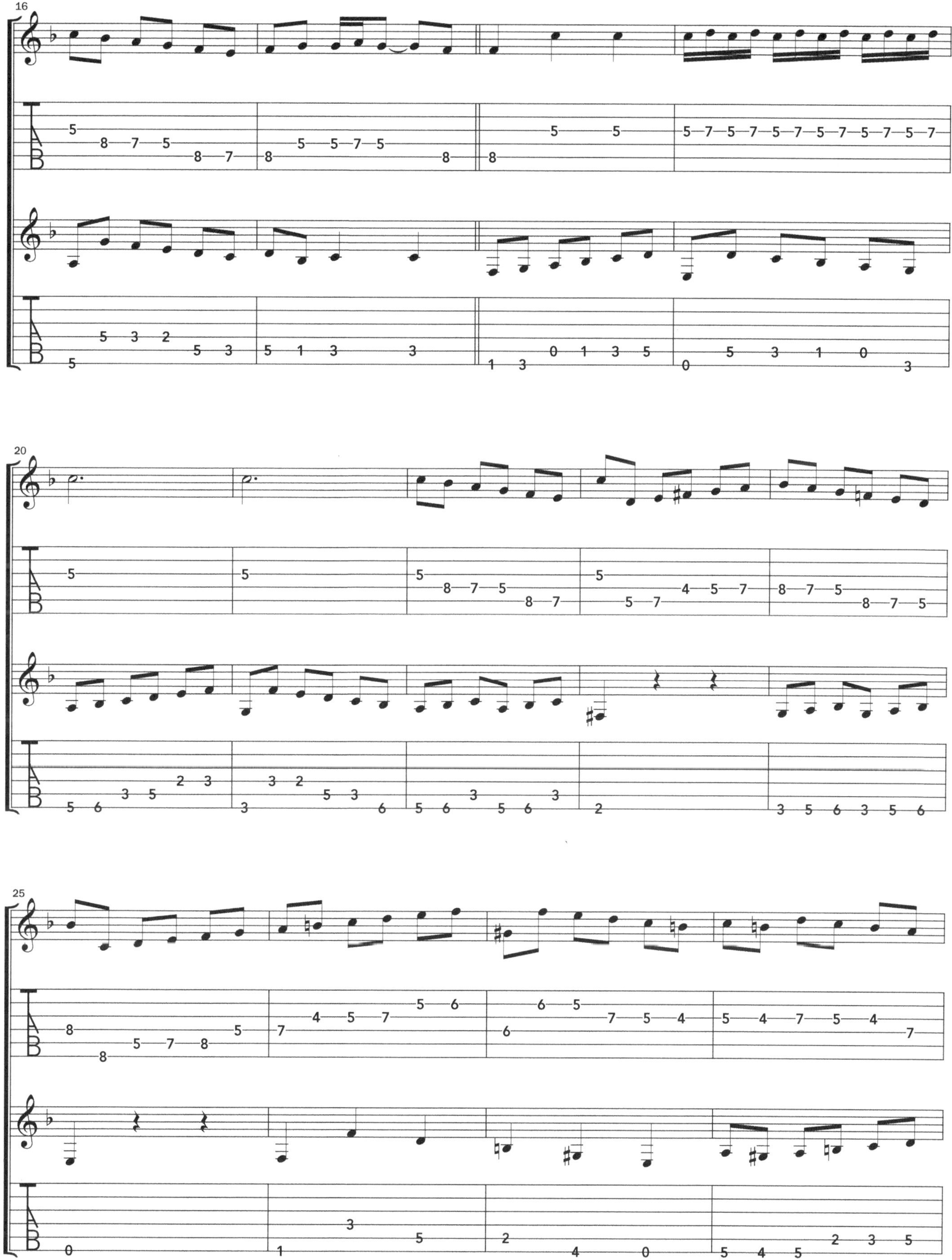
16
20
25

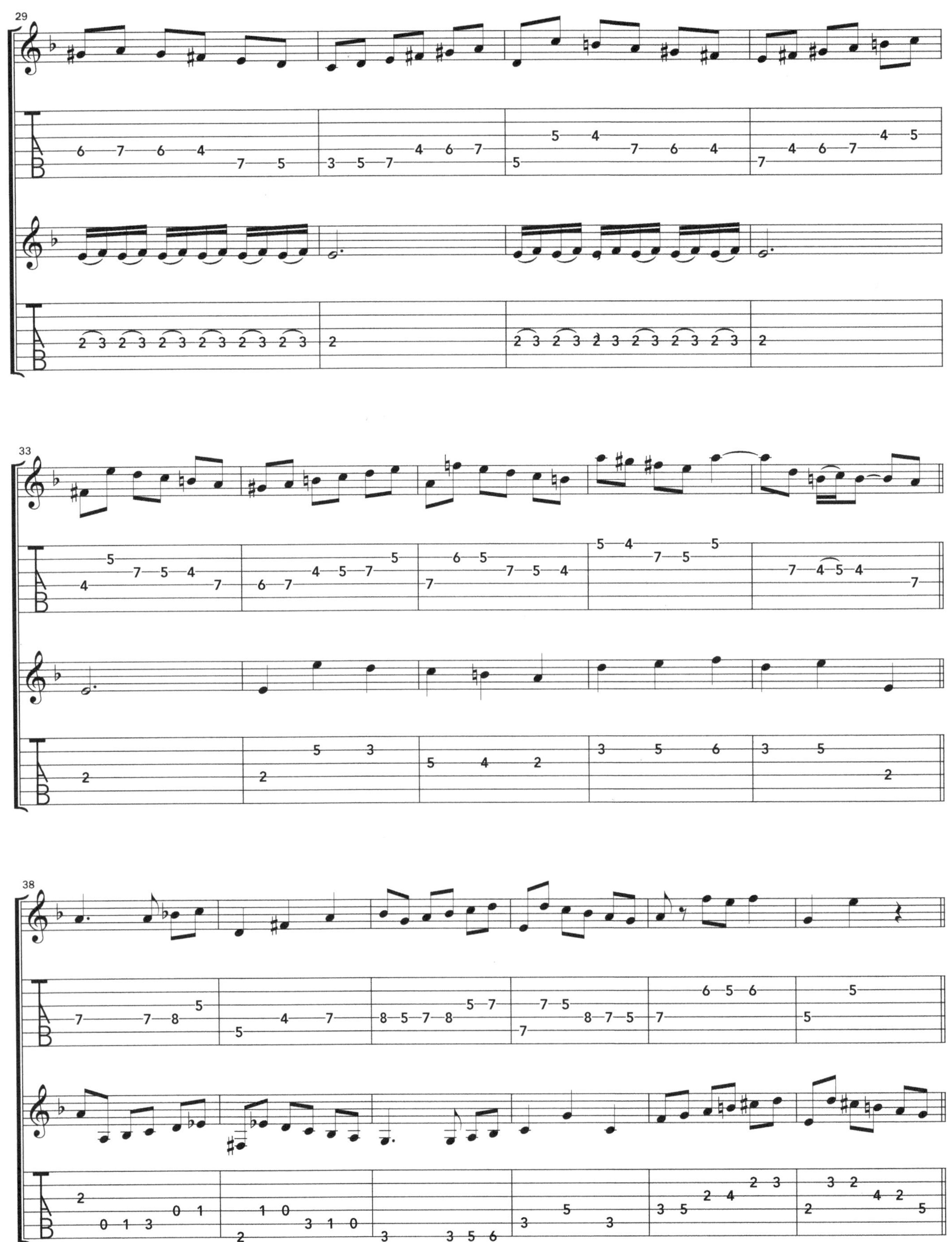

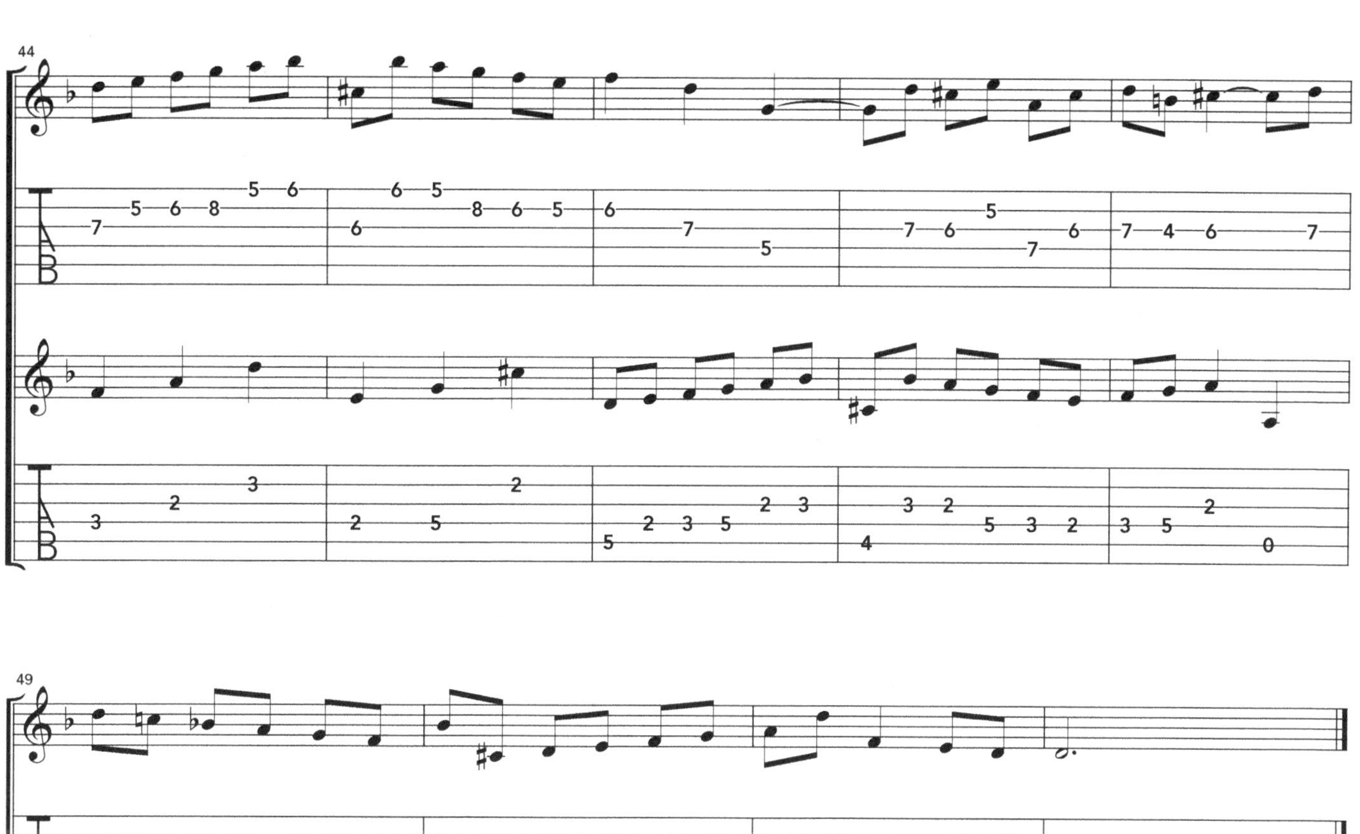
44

Example 39: Prelude to *Cello Suite No. 1* by J.S. Bach

Tuning: C G D G B E

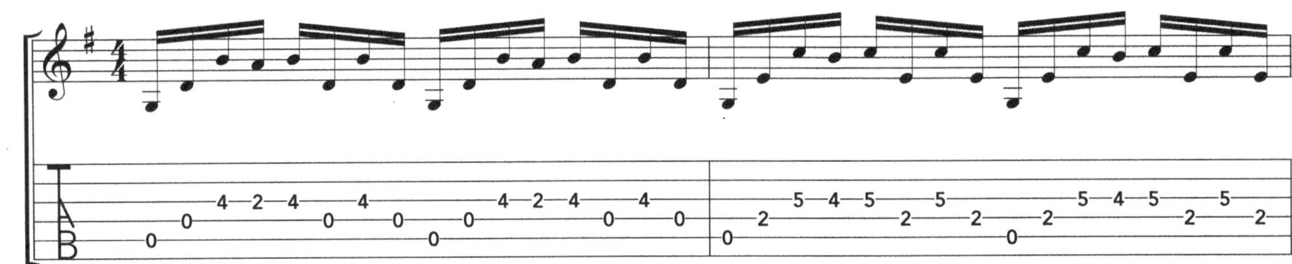

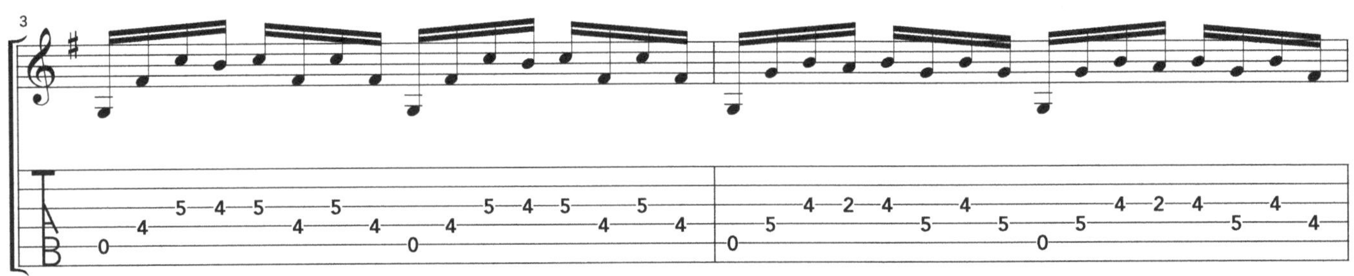

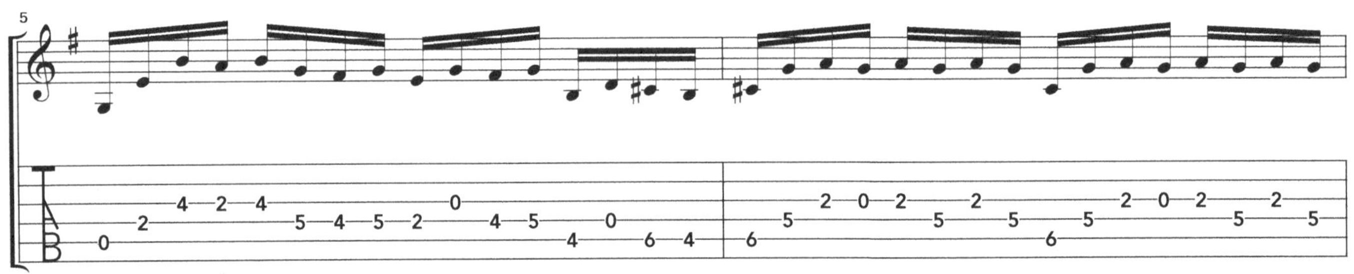

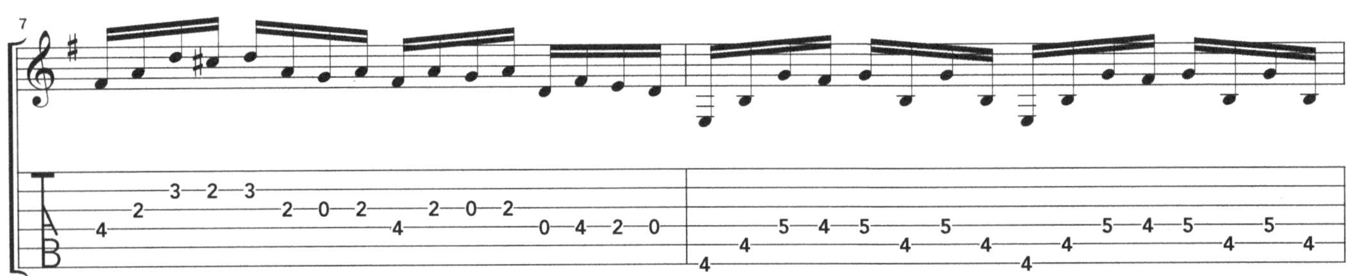

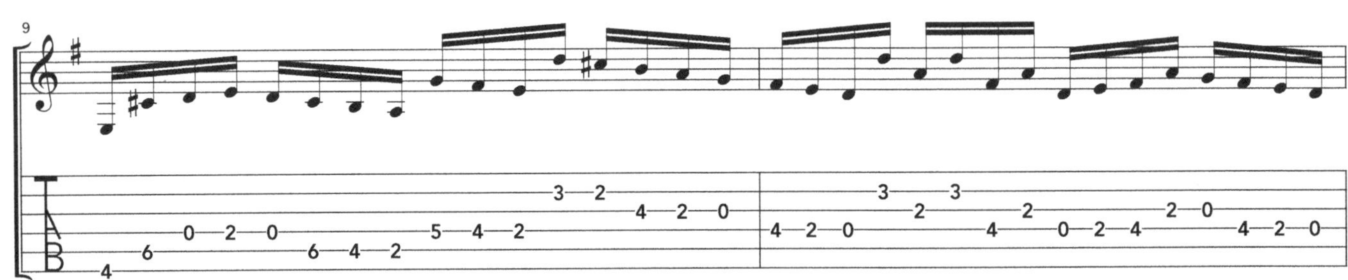

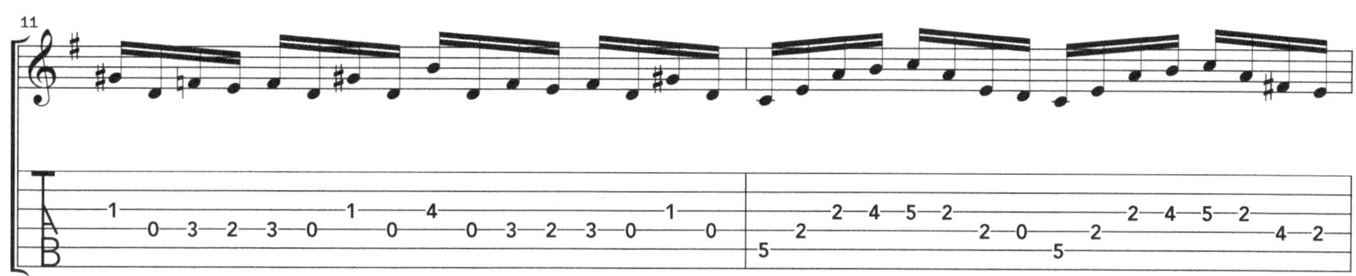

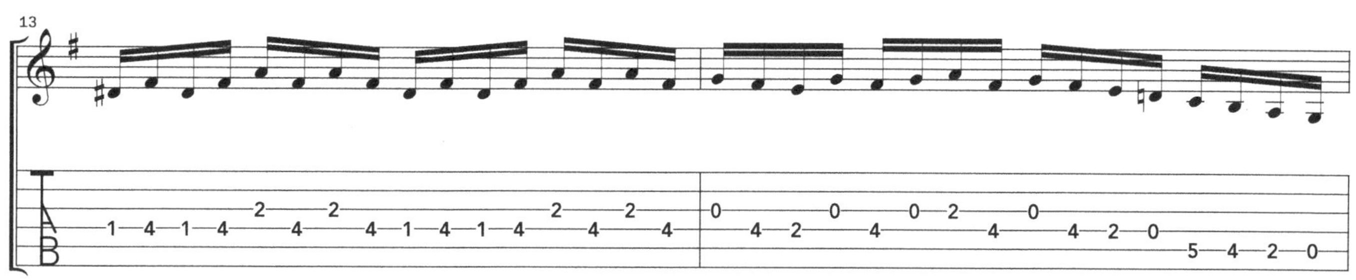

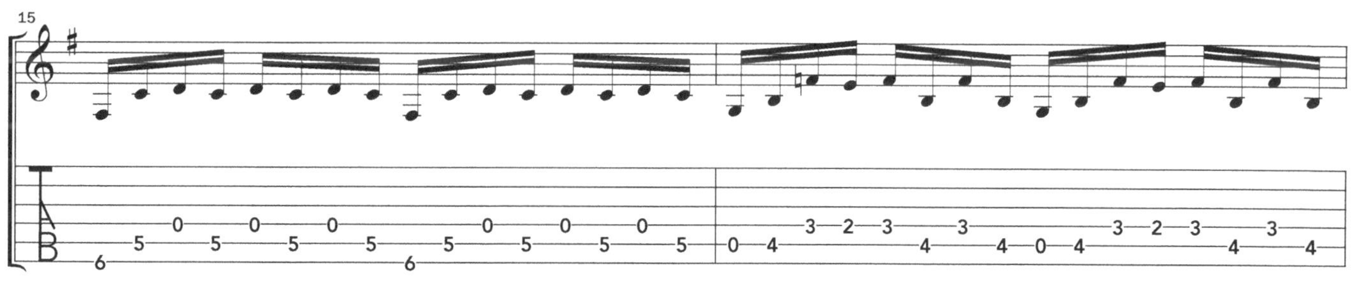

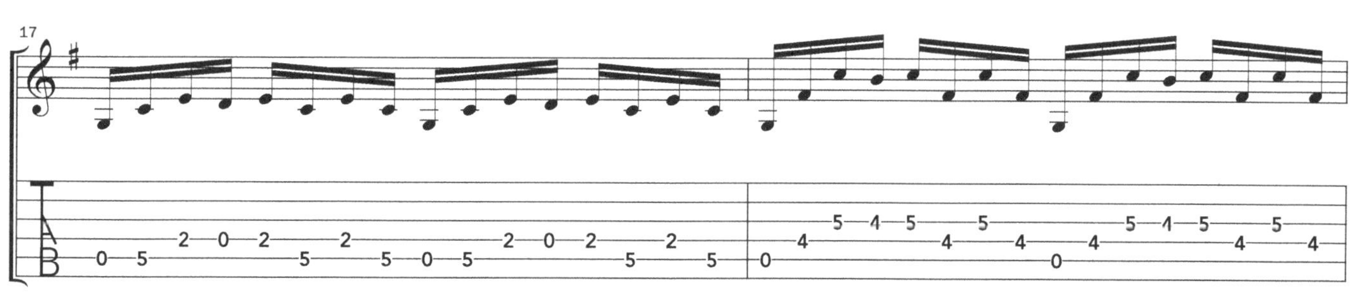

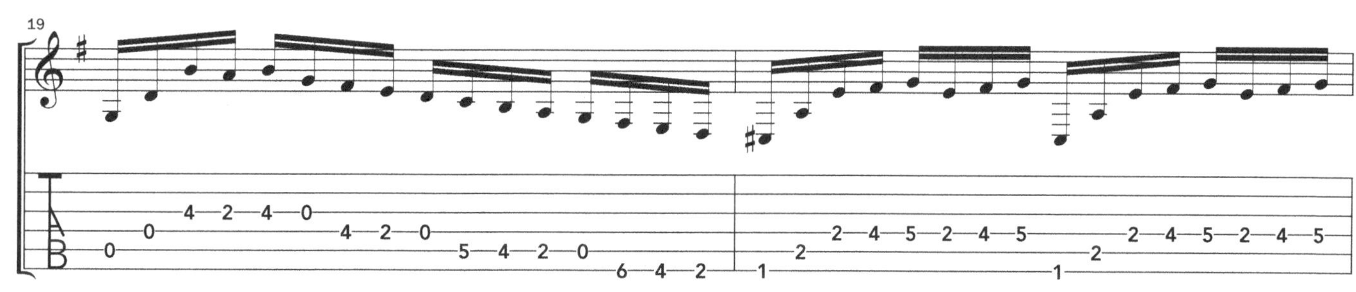

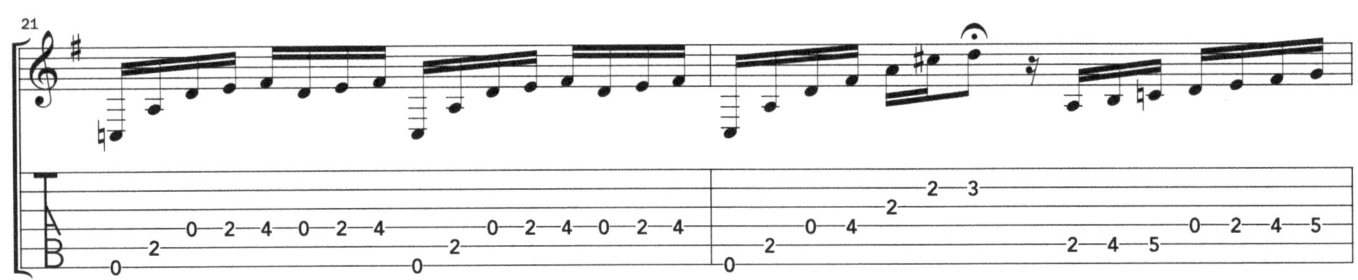
21

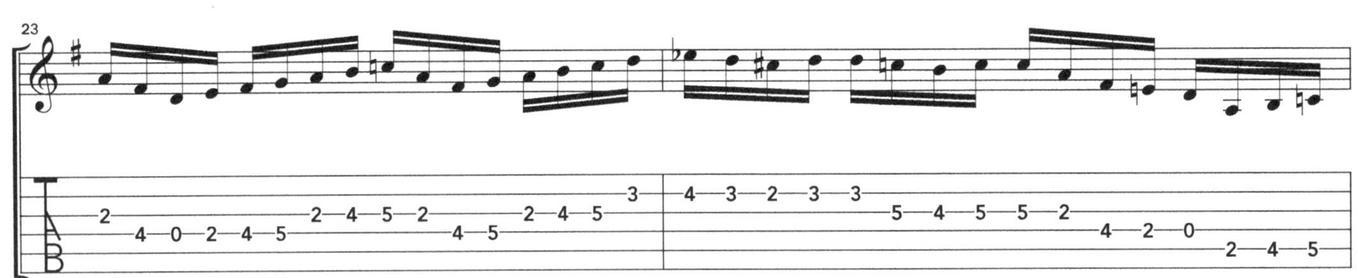
23

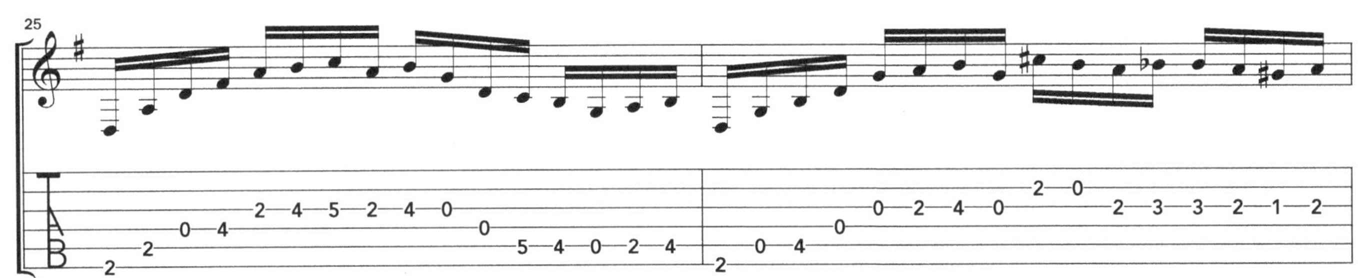
25

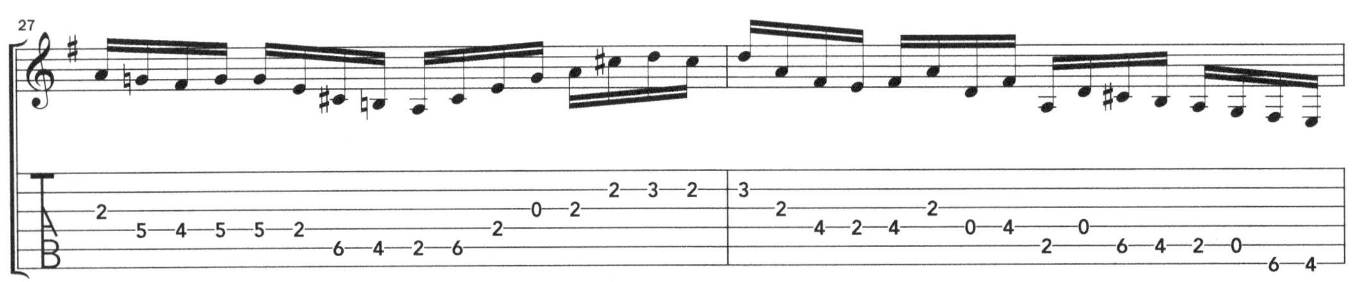
27

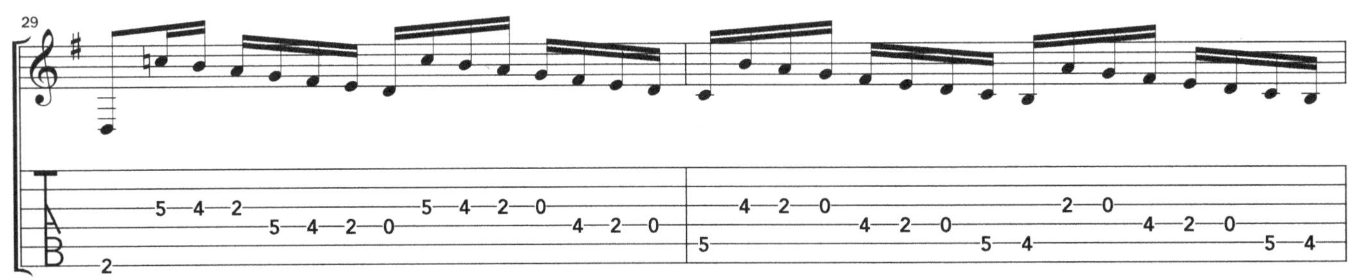
29

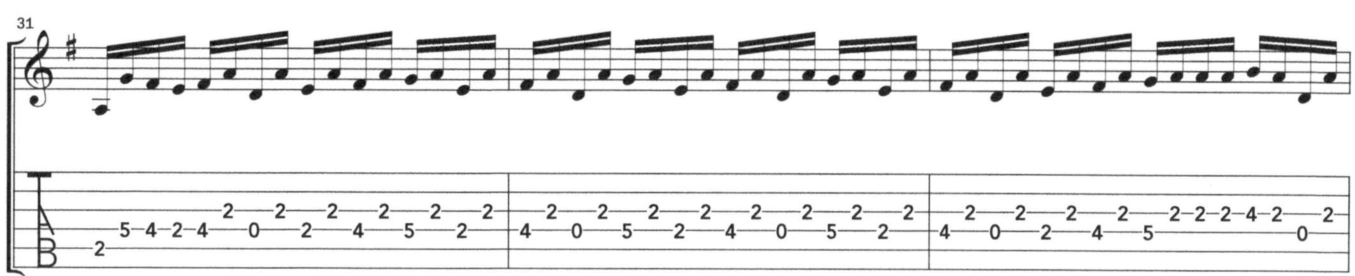
31
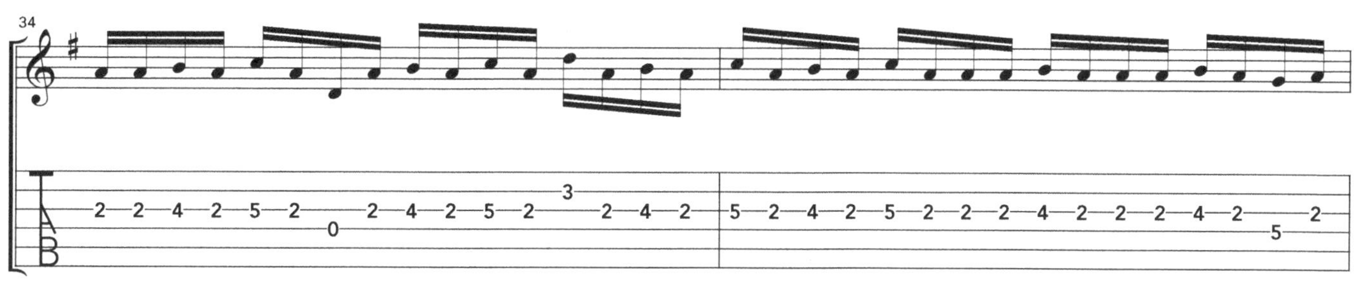
34
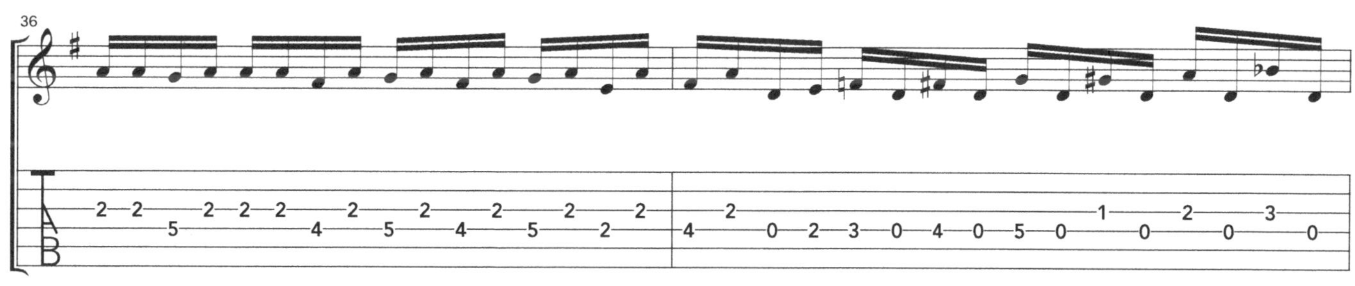
36
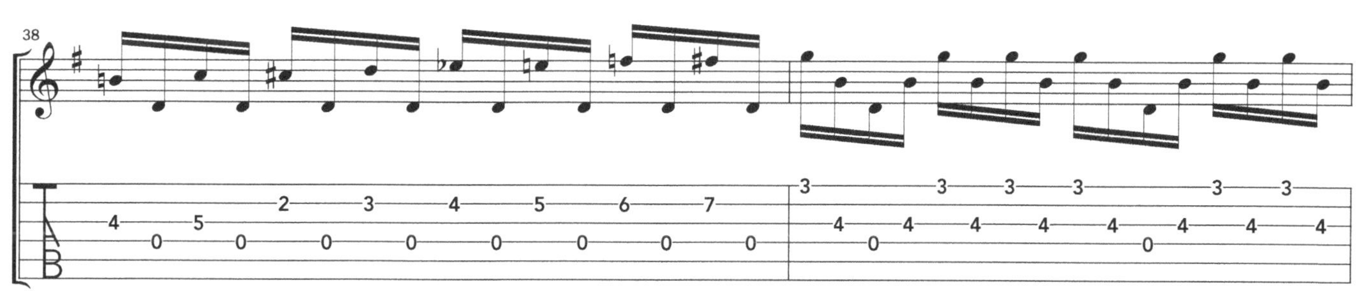
38
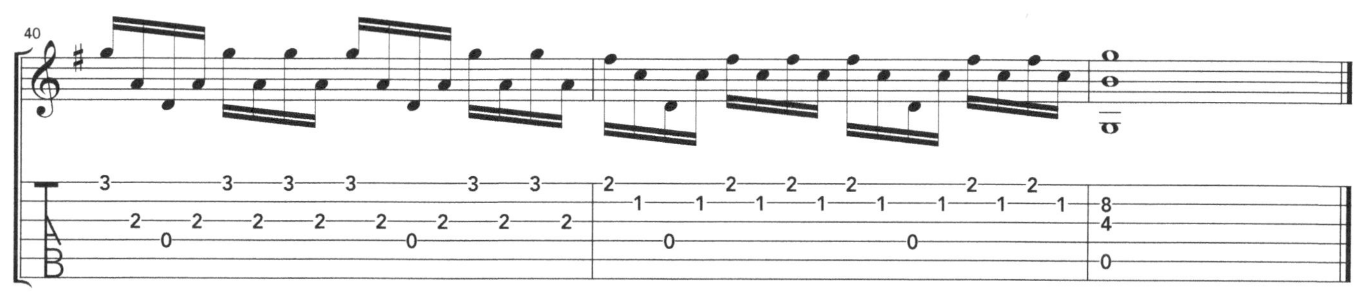
40

CHAPTER SEVEN

Creative Practicing
Part One

"Nulla dies sine linea—Not a day without a line"
–PLINY THE ELDER

The above quote from Roman scholar and naturalist Gaius Plinius Secundus—also known as Pliny the Elder—is often used in the context of practicing something every day, consistently, without necessarily considering the results or outcome. Instead, the focus is on the consistency of the process. His statement was originally in reference to the ancient Greek painter Apelles, who reportedly didn't let a day pass without at least drawing a line. Generations of artists and writers have used this and other quotes for inspiration. In short: Just do the work.

Some guitarists swear by a disciplined routine, while others play regularly, even if they don't necessarily practice in a structured way. Others say that they're thinking about music even if they don't have a guitar on hand. Jazz guitarist Wes Montgomery once said, "I'm putting hard efforts into [playing guitar]—this is where people have been mistaken about me. They don't know about the times when I'd be sitting up, just thinking. If I'd go to a movie show, I'd be looking at the picture, but I'd be hearing changes. You understand? This is how much determination I had for playing."

In his book *The Pierre Bensusan Guitar Collection*, the guitarist writes, "I play as often as I can. When I do not play, I sing, whistle, drum my hands on the table, walk in rhythm, write, teach music, talk about it, listen to it, dream about it… daily exercises, as well as an exciting repertoire and techniques, are essential to help us stay connected and keep enjoying practicing."

The bottom line is that playing guitar is always a good thing to do. However, those of us who have felt creatively stifled or frustrated by stagnation can benefit from a consistent practice routine, which should also include playing for pure enjoyment. Like any healthy habit, getting into the groove of a regular practice routine may take a minute, but you will be rewarded by growth and fulfillment.

Prelude No. 7

Gadd9
Dm7(♭6)
Gmaj9
Dm7(♭6)
Gadd9
Cm7(♭6)
C6/9♯11
F13sus4
F13♯11
Dm7(♭6)
Em11
Am9
Bm7
Fmaj9
Bm7
A6/9 /E
Gmaj7♯11
Dm7(♭6)
Gmaj13
Dm7(♭6)
Gmaj13
Dm7(♭6)
E6/9
art. harm.

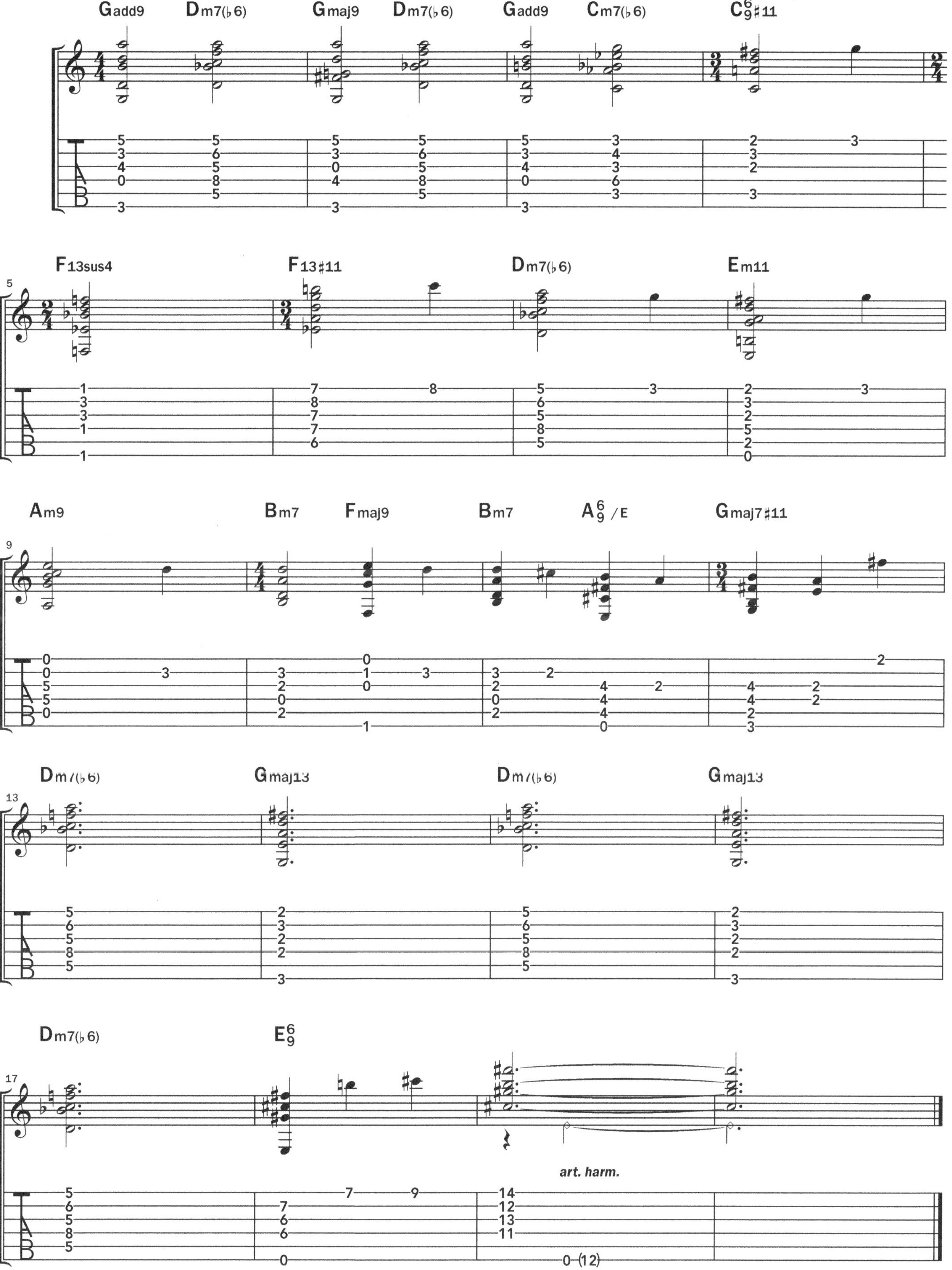

Types of Practice

Of course, there are many different types of practice and ways to organize your practice sessions, depending on the desired outcome, e.g., an upcoming performance, specific guitar and musical goals, or nurturing your creative muse. To keep your routine fresh, mix up the elements of practice, some with specific objectives and others focused on the satisfaction of playing. Below are some ideas about exploring different types of practice, followed by three stages of learning.

Repertoire

Learning, revisiting, and perfecting repertoire typically dominate practice sessions, and for good reason. Whether you are preparing for an upcoming concert or tour, or learning new music for your own enjoyment, practicing repertoire is the best overall way to develop technique, dynamics, musical delivery, and understanding of melody, harmony, and rhythm.

One way to be efficient with your practice time is to isolate and work on technically challenging song sections. Some classical pieces, for instance, have accompanying études or excerpts that focus on a particularly demanding technique. Indeed, many of J.S. Bach's celebrated works were originally composed as études for his students. Technical isolation exercises—such as those that strengthen the fretting hand and develop picking-hand fluidity—will certainly help, but nothing can replace working on actual music, which is why bebop players or flatpickers practice Charlie Parker melodies, Bud Powell melodies, or fiddle tunes to develop their ability to play quick tempos.

After you have practiced a passage to the point where you can play it flawlessly at (or just under) tempo, put it back in context and practice getting in and out of the passage. During isolation, of course, practice slowly to make sure your hands and ears—and most importantly, your mind—absorbs it. Follow up your practice with visualizations in which you see, hear, and feel the music in your mind. This will reinforce your knowledge of the music and give you the best odds of playing it perfectly in performance.

Once you have a solid mastery of the technical aspects and can play a complete passage from memory, focus on dynamics, flow, tempo, groove, and articulation to make it sound musical. That may sound like an ineffable term, but emotions, touch, interpretation, time-feel, tone production, nuance, delivery, and confidence all help the listener experience something special when you play.

Visual/Emotional/Artistic

Focusing on things other than the actual music—improvising on a particular feeling, or visual and literary prompts, for example—is another way to develop a soulful presentation of music. Imagine someone is reading a story or poem and you are providing the musical soundtrack. What would that sound like? What would that feel like?

Early in my performing career, I had the opportunity to do this with a modern dance company. It was incredibly refreshing, initially challenging, and ultimately very rewarding. There were no musical cues per se ("Play softer! Do a blues run! Keep a vamp going in E Lydian!"); it was all based on intuition, as well as timing and certain physical cues that were worked out in advance. But it was entirely up to me to score the choreography, and rarely have I felt so connected to my guitar.

Many guitarists like to score visuals by playing along to the many silent YouTube videos that show nature, landscapes, travel, special effects, etc. You could watch almost anything, turn down the sound, and play what you experience visually and emotionally. This type of practice is a great way to develop your musicality.

Try improvising some music in response to this image.

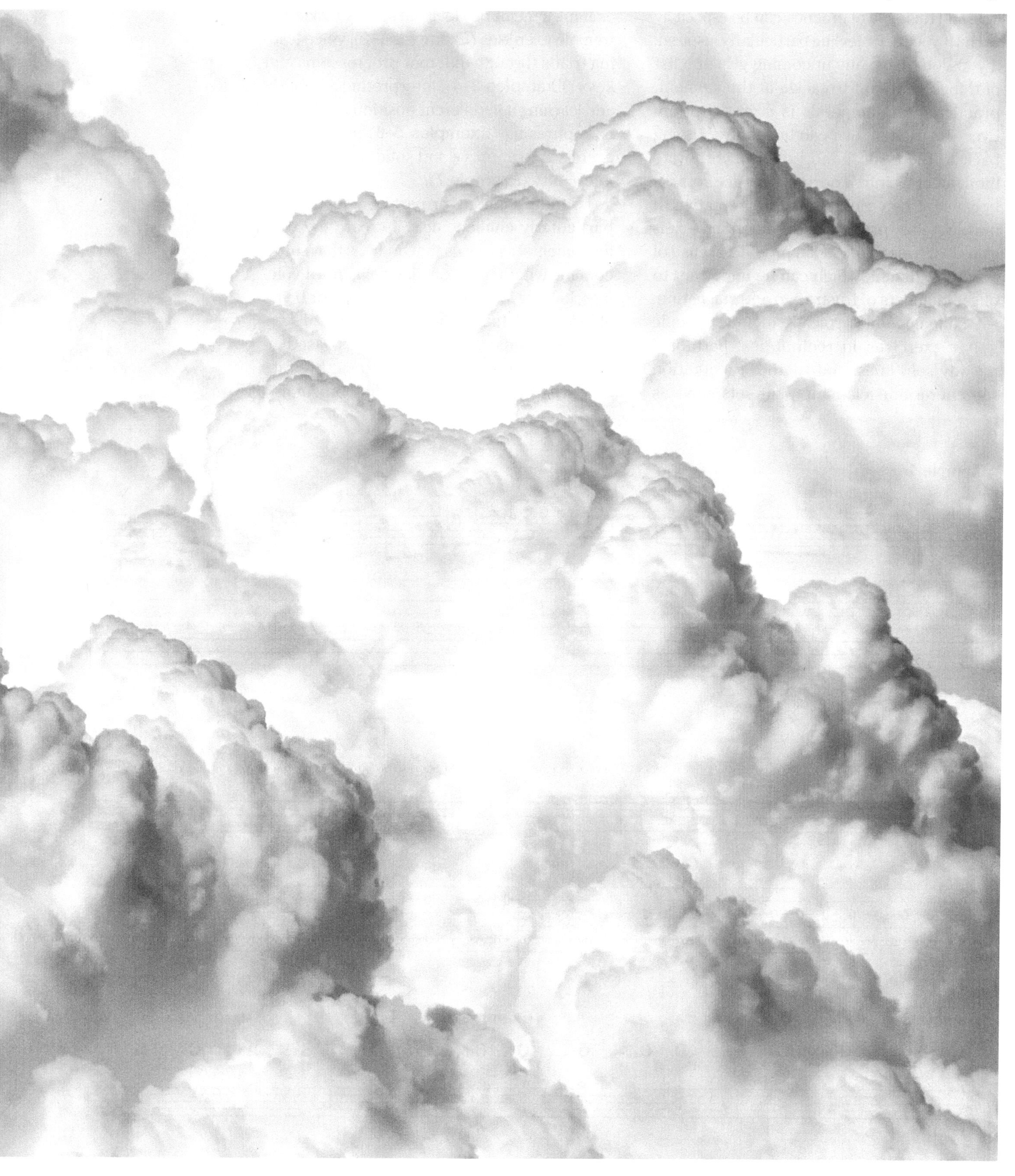

Fundamentals of Guitar Technique

It's always a good time to practice fundamentals, and this type of practice can be especially useful if you're not feeling particularly inspired. If you don't have any upcoming gigs or a list of things you want to tackle at the moment, practicing fundamentals is a great option. Every instrumentalist can benefit from going back to the basics, and I often incorporate fundamentals into a normal practice session because it can yield something creative. If nothing else, practicing rudimentary exercises just feels good. It can provide a sense of accomplishment, which can be important to offset moments of frustration and stagnation.

Fundamentals typically include specific guitar exercises in techniques, harmony, melody/solo lines, and rhythm (in addition to general musicianship skill sets such as reading, ear-training, study of concepts). Some examples might be slow and steady picking or tremolo exercises (**Examples 1–2**), voice-leading triads through different progressions and keys (**Examples 3–4**), interpreting a melody and learning it in different positions with alternate phrasing (**Examples 5–6**), and playing exercises to improve and solidify your rhythmic acuity (**Example 7**).

If there's a song or part of a song that's particularly challenging, I'll create my own fundamental exercises that address that shortcoming, whether it's playing new chord voicings, locking into a particular groove, or being able to pick steady eighth notes at a blisteringly fast tempo. Creating exercises based on your goals can be a great way to incorporate creativity into the practice of fundamentals.

Example 1

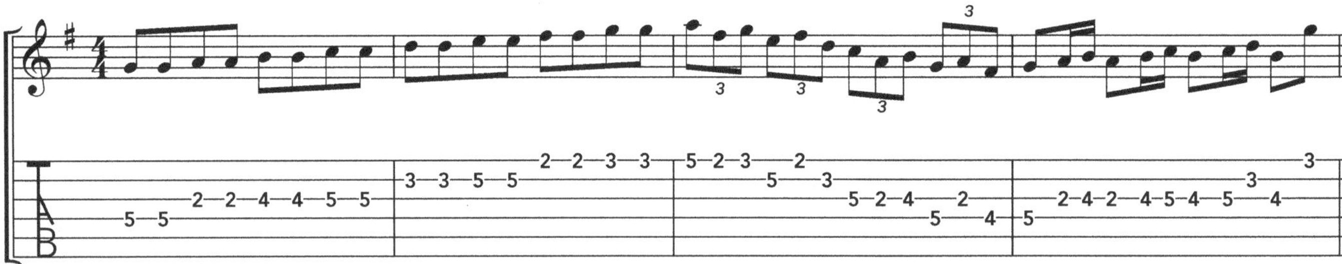

Example 2

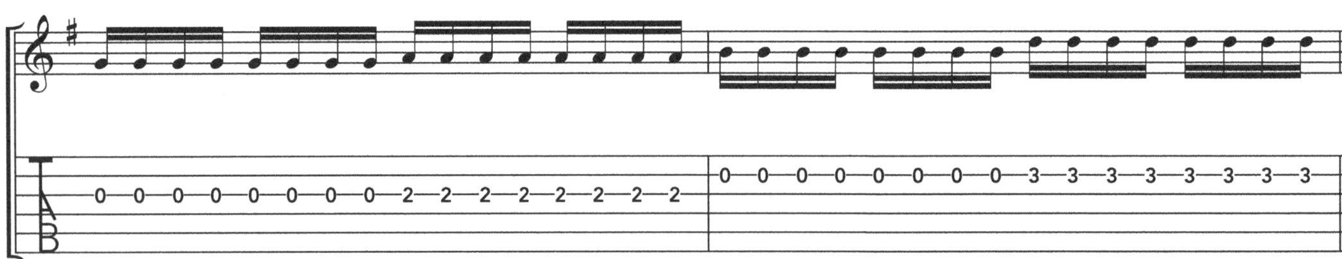

Example 3 **Example 4**

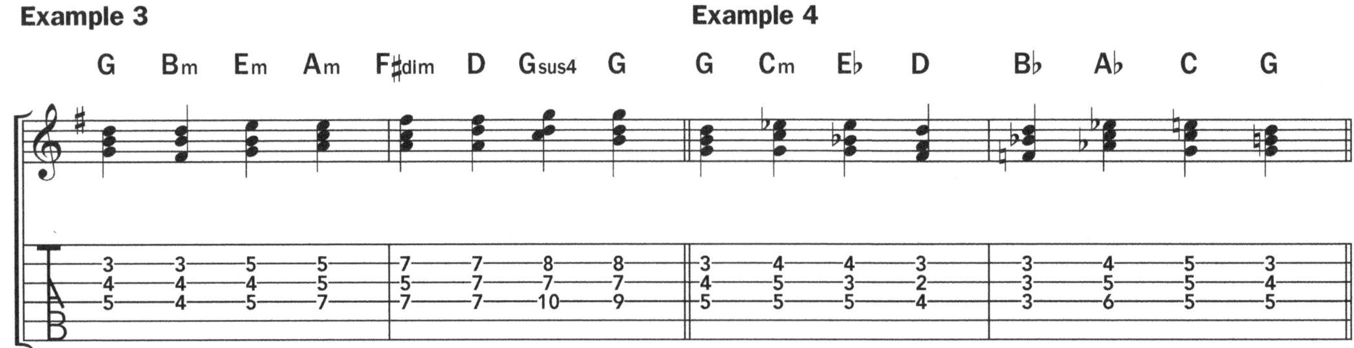

Example 5

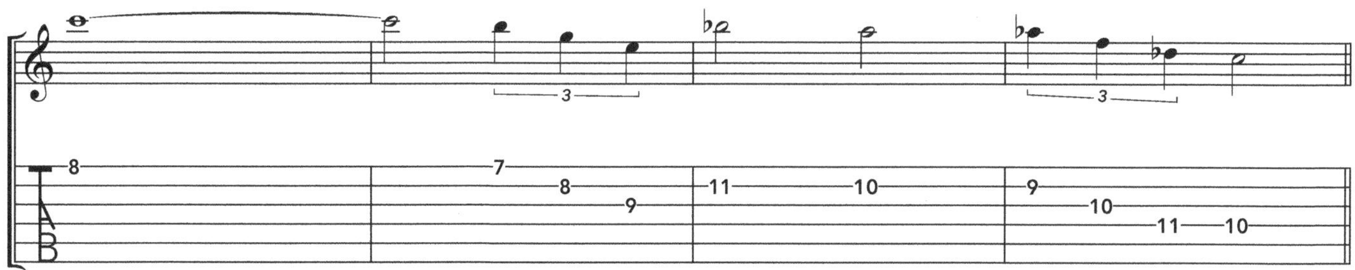

Example 6

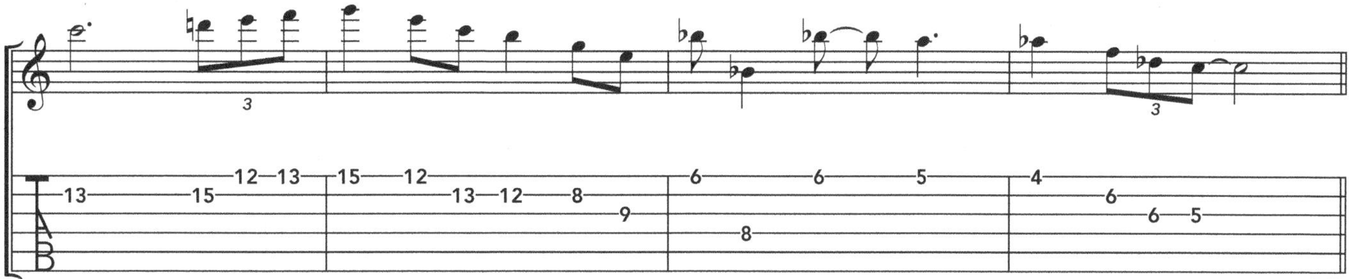

Example 7

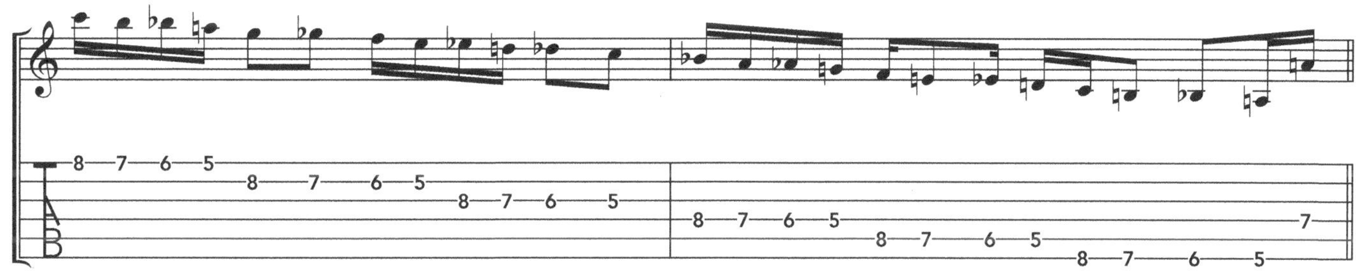

Musical Skill Sets

I consider these to be universal musicianship skills that are often (but not always) acquired through formal study. Musical literacy would include the ability to read music, as well as the ability to hear deeply, transcribe, and learn music by ear. Transcribing and analysis are powerful tools when learning about a particular genre or diving deep into a favorite player, especially in one's formative stages. Everyone starts out with heavy influences and spends a significant amount of time trying to emulate what it is that attracts them to that player. Doing this up to a certain point can be tremendously beneficial, as it presents different perspectives, ideas, and approaches. Learning solos and music from other guitarists—and especially other singers and instrumentalists—can give you ample ideas to create your own style.

If you are a professional guitarist, expanding upon your musical skill sets is a good way to increase employment opportunities. Many guitarists will double on other instruments, for example, or are proficient with recording equipment, musical direction, arranging, composing, or transcription.

Composing and Arranging

For many guitarists, writing and arranging music play a significant role in their musical identity and aspirations. Even if you don't consider yourself a composer, developing your own arrangements of cover songs does wonders for your knowledge of harmony, form, melody, and counterpoint. The process of composing is very personal. A common question in masterclasses is, "Which comes first, the melody or chord progression?" This is something of a chicken-and-egg conundrum. Personally, I believe there are numerous ways of approaching composition. Sometimes the muse hits and, if we're lucky, a complete song will reveal itself out of nowhere.

In other cases, you can spend weeks, months, or even years working on a particular tune. Most writers have a ton of half-completed songs hanging around, either written or recorded, and sometimes it can take a while to write the perfect bridge, chorus, or ending to a song that needs finishing.

Some writers are deeply inspired by the process of co-writing with other musicians. Accountability is an added bonus of collaborating, and truly, nothing inspires quite like a looming deadline. In my experience, it's helpful to have a treasure trove of harmonic, stylistic, and theoretical knowledge. You can start writing from an inspired idea or feeling, and if you get stuck, you can use your knowledge of music. The best way to solve a musical problem is to ask musical questions: "What would it sound like if I used this harmonic device? Should the time-feel change? Maybe even a time signature change? Should it modulate?" Continuing to ask "what-if" questions with an open sense of curiosity will always invite creative solutions.

Anything Goes

Sometimes, it's important to just play. I like to fold this element into a regular session anyway, usually at the end, right before a cool-down. You may choose to revisit challenging material from earlier in the session or week, play an old favorite song, improvise to tracks, or just play freestyle. It's your call. Doing this every so often is not only beneficial, but therapeutic.

Another thing you can do, which is often overlooked, is to play along with a favorite recording. You don't need to worry about getting every single note correct, as you would with an academic transcription. It's more about tapping into the groove, the overall vibe, and the intensity of the performance. Don't worry about the notes—focus on the groove and feeling of the song.

Jam Sessions and Playing with Others

Playing music with others is one of the most beneficial forms of practice and can teach us important lessons in real time. Jam sessions are time-honored traditions and special community gatherings where like-minded people of all ages and abilities learn to play music together, and I've always required my guitar students at the University of Colorado Denver to attend at least one jazz jam session per semester. Stepping onstage to play with other musicians you don't know can be daunting, but learning etiquette, musical exchange, how to listen and support, what to play, and what not to play simply cannot be replicated during solitary practice or even in applied lessons.

Three Stages of Learning

Discovery, Creative Exploration, and Mastery

Drawing from my years as a practicing musician and educator, I've observed that there are three distinct stages of learning and practice. I refer to these stages as discovery, creative exploration, and mastery, and while they do occur in this sequence, they also overlap, much like a Venn diagram. Let's take a closer look at how to progress at each stage.

The first stage is discovery. Things are sparkling and brand new, perhaps with the thrill of discovering a great new chord voicing or progression, mapping out a scale or arpeggio in a new area of the fretboard, studying theory, or learning a new tune. Entirely new concepts may feel a bit overwhelming, but we begin practicing even if we don't fully understand it all quite yet. This is the shortest of the three stages.

After learning something for the first time, the next stage involves practicing and exploring these new ideas. This is where we live most of the time. Growth and fresh perspectives continue indefinitely, and revisiting material you didn't fully understand at first helps it make perfect sense. This stage is what I refer to as creative exploration, and the word "creative" is intentional. There's always a way to be creative and enjoy the process even if you're learning or practicing seemingly stale concepts.

Not only is it important to be creative, but also efficient. For example: To avoid wasting time, try to practice several things simultaneously. As a rule of thumb, I'll add an element of rhythm (using the metronome whenever possible) and technique to whatever concept I'm practicing (e.g., a new scale pattern). I'm still essentially practicing the main concept, but I'm also working on additional aspects. On top of this, I'll incorporate the element of creativity by improvising and literally playing with the material.

The third stage is what I consider mastery. I don't use this term in an esoteric sense or from the standpoint of finally reaching a seemingly unattainable goal. To me, mastery simply means that in the context of playing, composing, performing—whatever it is—you're able to use material you've been gradually developing. We are constantly building our musical vocabulary, making new and challenging concepts an organic part of our playing, and when these concepts are immediately accessible without having to think about them, that's mastery!

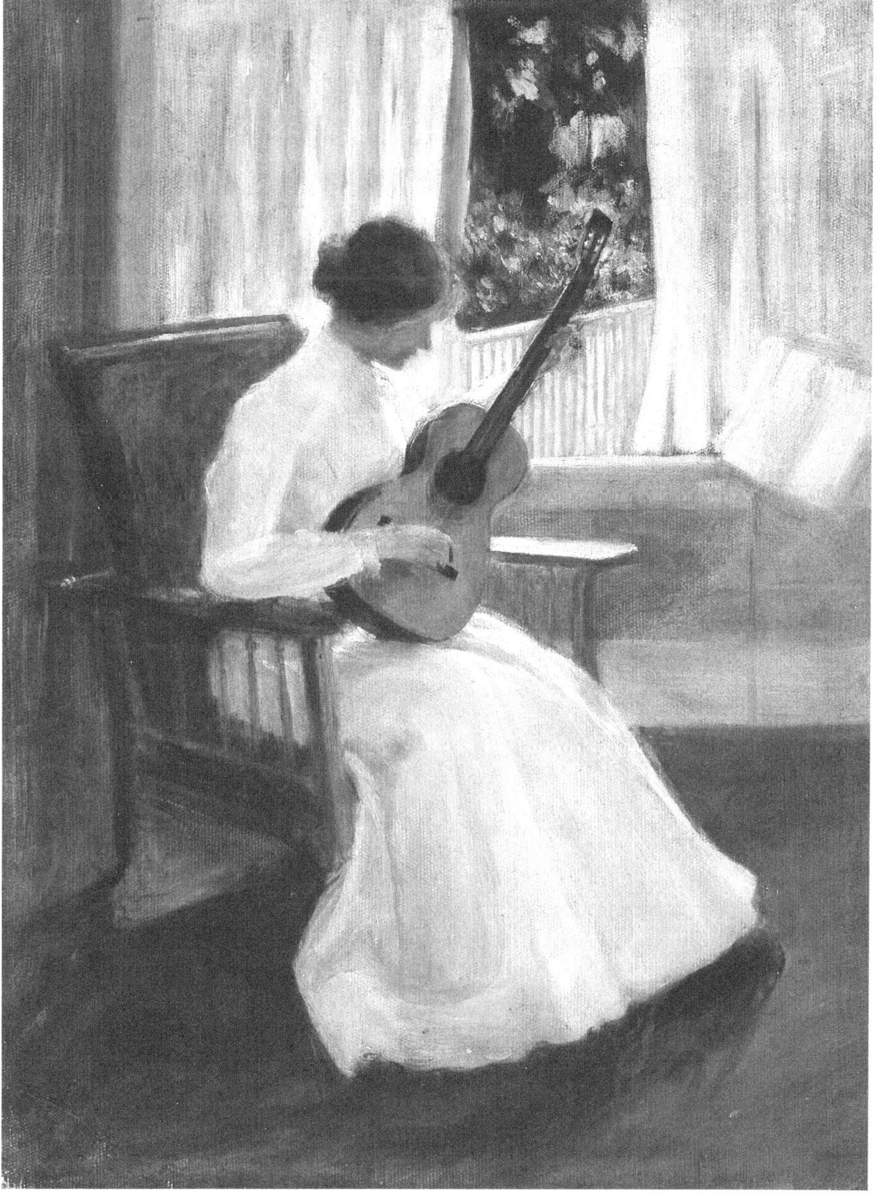

KATE CLIFTON OSGOOD HOLMES, SUMMER, 1903

Now let's put this into action with a few examples. Let's say we are learning the basic G major scale pattern in **Example 8**. In this case, the discovery phase is simply getting our fingers in the right place, coordinating with the picking hand to play the notes, and eventually committing the pattern to memory. Of course, we have a great advantage with the transposing nature of the guitar—once you learn that G major pattern, you can move it up two frets to play A major, etc.

Once you've played through the pattern to the point where you have memorized or at least have a fair grasp on the subject, it's time for the creative exploration phase. As mentioned earlier, the objective here is to learn and practice the subject by having fun and being creative with the process.

After learning the basic scale pattern in Ex. 8, most guitarists would practice that same pattern using the same fingering, almost always starting with the root and playing ascending and descending. And they'll practice scales in that way forever! Now, there's nothing wrong with playing familiar patterns and using exercises for technique-building, but our goal is to explore and ultimately master the subject. The way to do that is by looking at the subject from several perspectives.

While working on the subject, let's incorporate some kind of technique and some kind of rhythm concept. **Example 9** still focuses on the same notes in the G major scale pattern, but it adds a technical focus (alternate picking) and a rhythmic element. **Example 10** takes the same G major scale and incorporates double-stops using a hybrid picking technique, plus quarter- and eighth-note triplets.

Example 11 illustrates a fun concept that is especially worthwhile for improvising guitarists. It uses question-and-answer between a solo line and the double-stop C to G figure on beats 3 and 4 of every other bar. Finally, **Example 12** features the same G major scale but in chordal figures mostly stacked in fourths, played on the offbeats of 1 and 3 while the metronome hits 2 and 4.

These examples show how one might explore a basic concept with the added benefit of technical and rhythmic elements. You can apply these principles to triads, arpeggios, chords, patterns, or any other subject; you can add techniques such as playing with the thumb, hybrid picking, fingerstyle, sweep or directional picking, or tapping; and you can add some type of rhythm exercise. And we all need to work on rhythm!

Example 8 **Example 9**

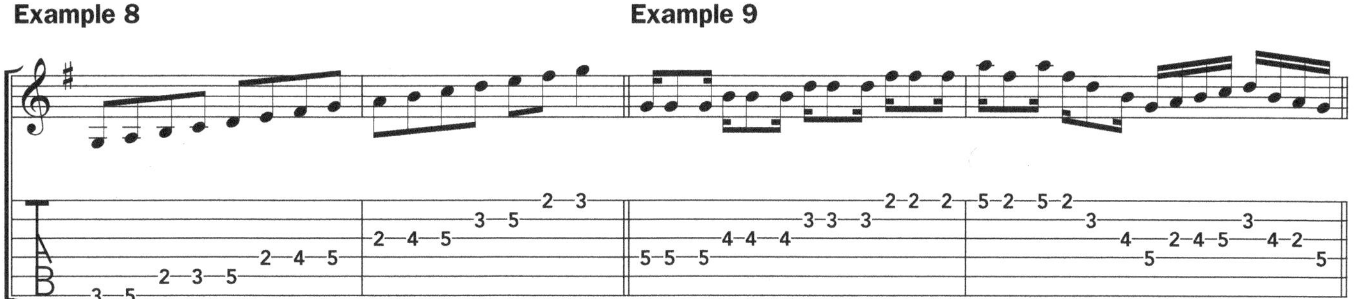

Example 10

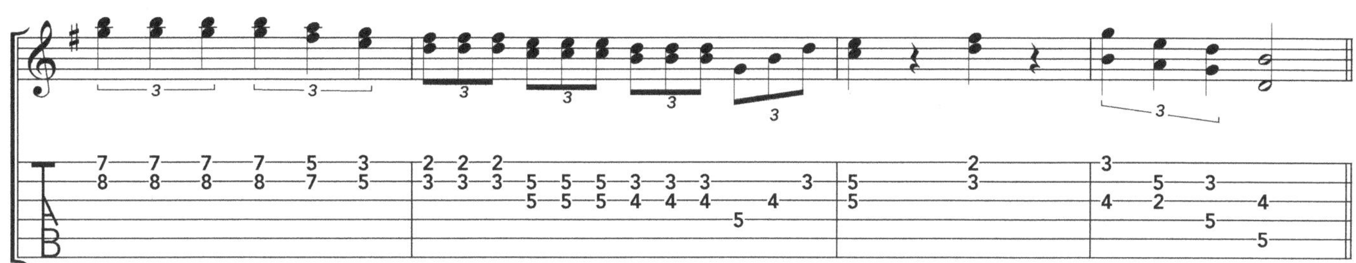

Example 11

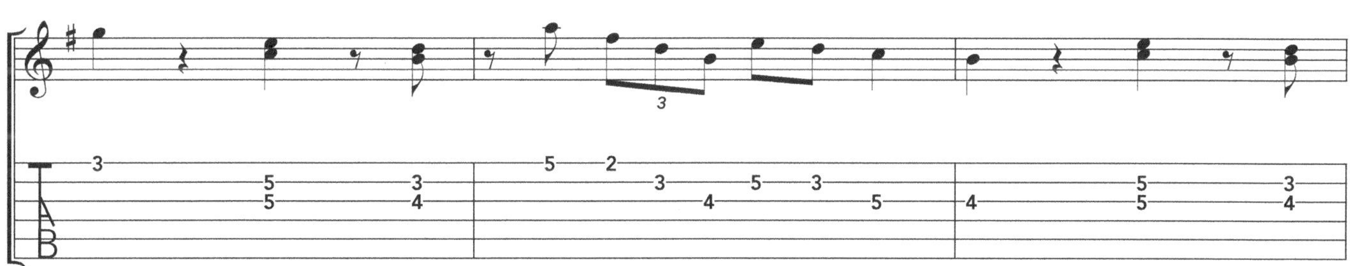

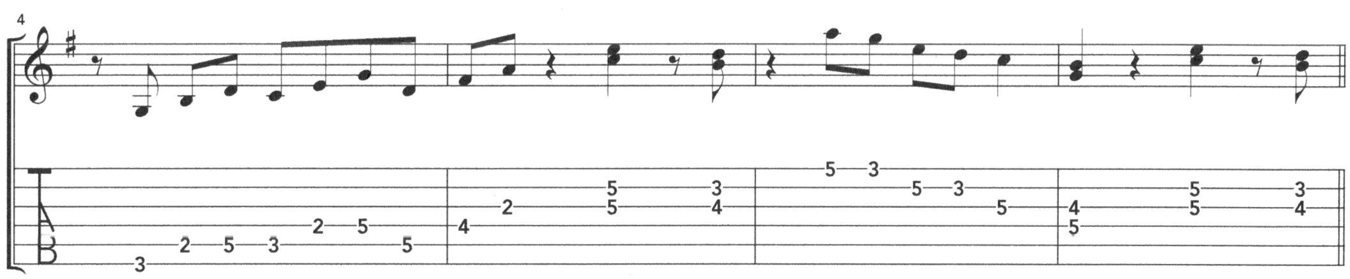

Example 12

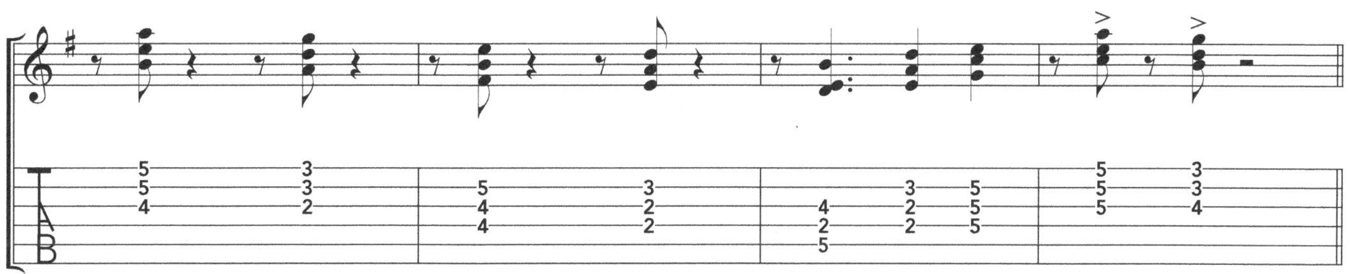

Set Limitations to Boost Creativity

Setting specific limitations can also enhance your creativity. By allowing yourself to only use certain fingers, techniques, string sets, positions, intervals, or rhythms, you are forced to use your ears and imagination; you won't be able to fall into stock fingerings or patterns you already know well. This is a common complaint among intermediate to advanced guitarists: They have worked so hard to learn all the theory, shapes, licks, and patterns, yet they feel they are just running the changes or playing the same old lines over and over. Setting limitations can immediately get you out of this rut and help foster creativity in the practice studio or onstage.

Practicing with limitations is like a creative game you can use when working on solo ideas. Let's return to the earlier concept of playing question and answer solo lines, where you play a melodic line question on the top two strings only, followed by a chordal answer. This effect works well when soloing over a blues (**Example 13**). You could also reverse this by playing solo lines on the bottom two strings, complemented by upper-register chord figures, as shown in **Example 14**.

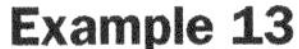

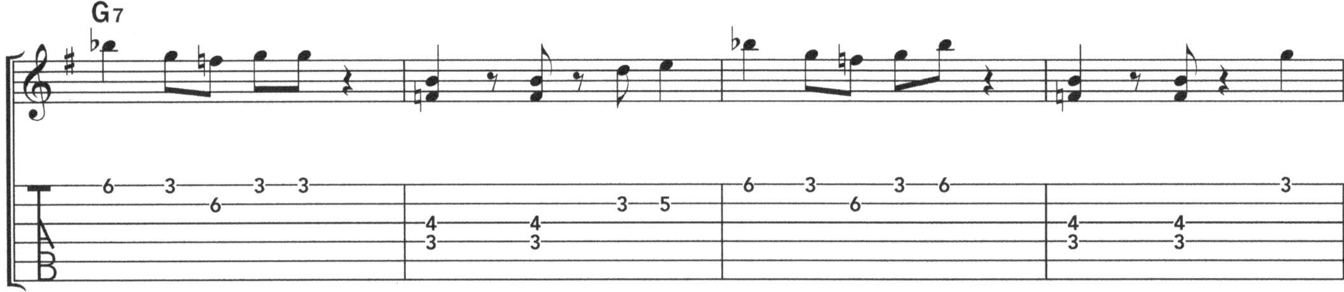

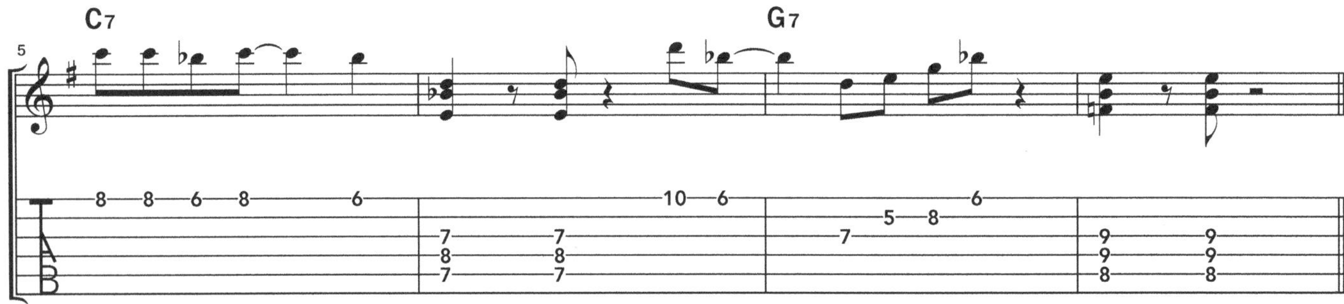

Example 14

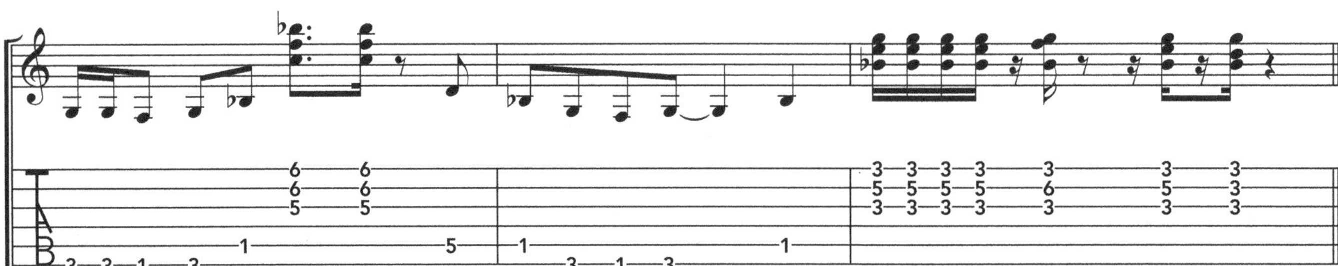

Playing with Dynamics, Rhythm, and Time

An important element sometimes overlooked by non-classical guitarists is detailed attention to dynamics. You can practice using dynamics by playing a piece of music at different levels, from soft to medium to loud, or by taking a simple riff such as the bluegrass banjo-inspired **Example 15**, adding crescendos and decrescendos for dramatic effect, and repeating the riff at three distinctly different volume levels.

Practicing with the metronome on beats 2 and 4 of the measure (**Example 16)** is also an excellent way to develop your time and rhythm sensibilities. Being comfortable with time will also help you feel secure onstage, and this simple exercise will help.

If feeling the time on the backbeats (or off-beats) is challenging, try this: Set the metronome at 70 bpm (beats per minute) and for every click, count out loud "two-four-two-four" lining up those counts with the metronome clicks. Then in the spaces between the clicks, count "one-three-one-three". Finally, count "one-two-three-four" with the two and four counts lining up with the clicks. This will help you feel the overall time and comfortably line up with the backbeats. (Imagine a hi-hat or snare drum playing on 2 and 4, as the actual tempo will be 140 bpm). Increase or decrease the tempo as necessary, and when you're ready, try playing a scale without turning the time around. If you have a metronome app on your phone that has a voice feature counting out each beat, that may be helpful. Otherwise, practice using a click without any accents.

Once this feels comfortable, try playing **Example 17**, which creates the effect of a walking bassline playing the first five bars of a 12-bar blues progression.

Example 15

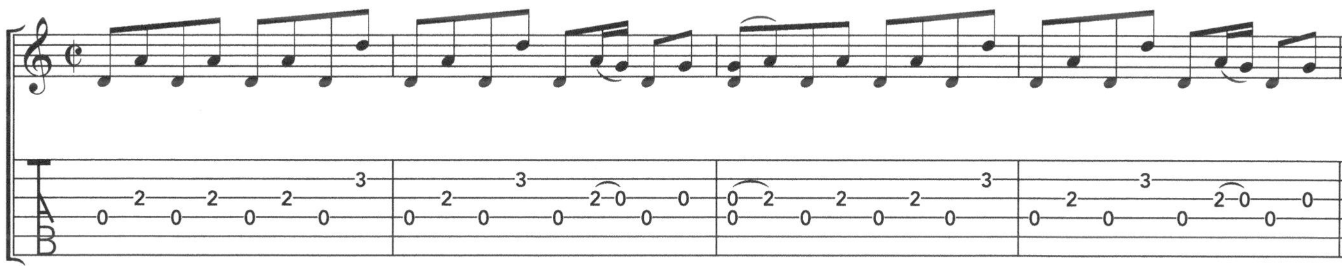

Example 16

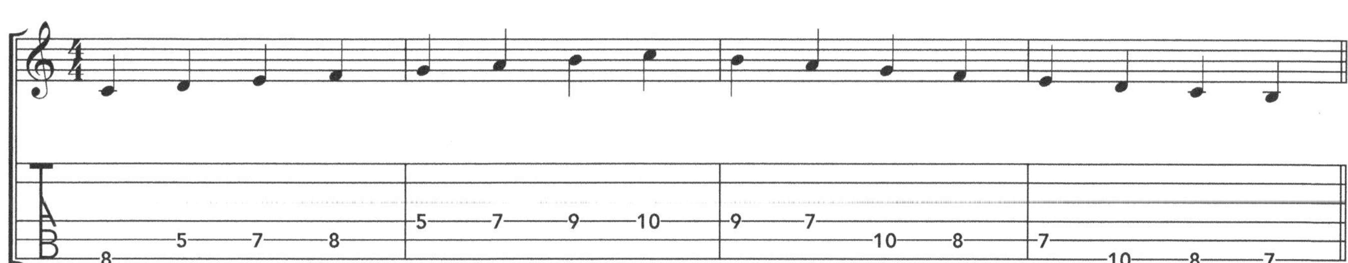

Example 17

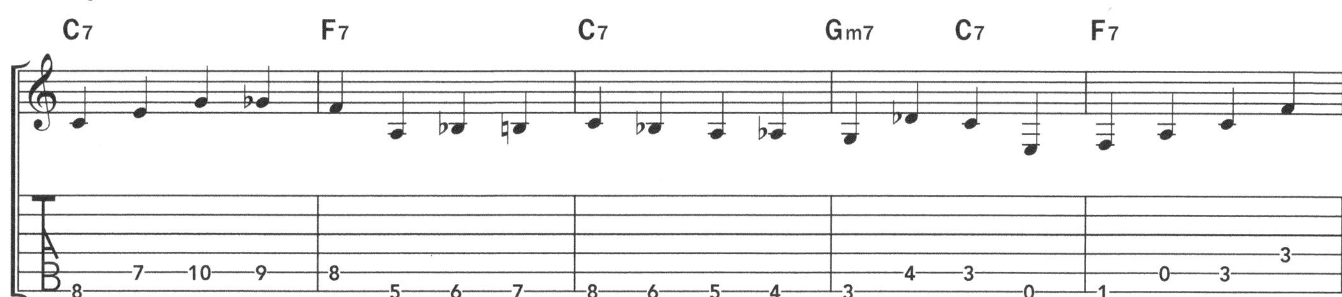

For more of a challenge, we can also have the metronome click on just one beat in a measure of 4/4 time. **Example 18** illustrates this with a blues shuffle riff in E. Set the metronome at 30 bpm (which would be an actual tempo of 120) and gradually line up with the beats using the same method as before. Start by counting "four" on the click, then double it up by adding a "two" and finally "one-two-three-four" with the click always sounding on beat four. This is a great exercise in subdividing the measure.

Another fun technique to explore is the use of cross-rhythms. In **Example 19**, we have a phrase (a quarter note followed by two eighth notes, tied to another quarter note) that lasts three beats and moves freely across the bar lines of 4/4 time. Using this cross-rhythm, also known as "three-against-four," can create a simple but wonderful polyrhythmic effect during solos or when writing guitar riffs. **Example 20** illustrates the same effect using a slightly different repeating rhythm with a chordal riff.

Example 18

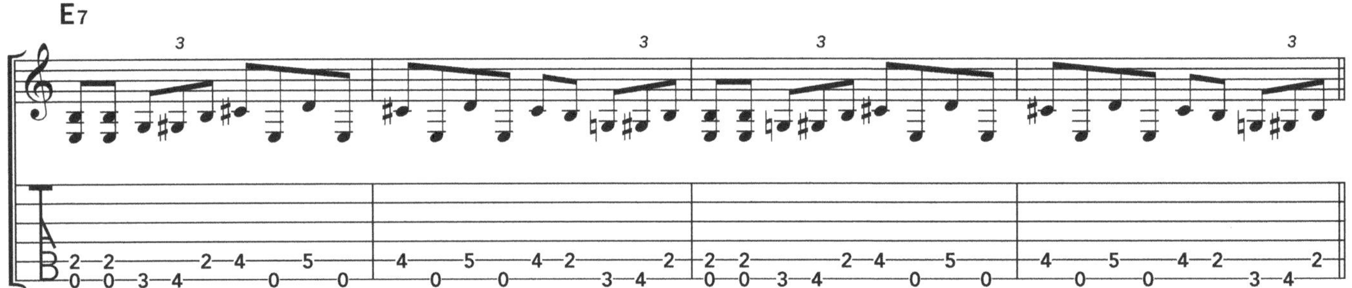

Example 19

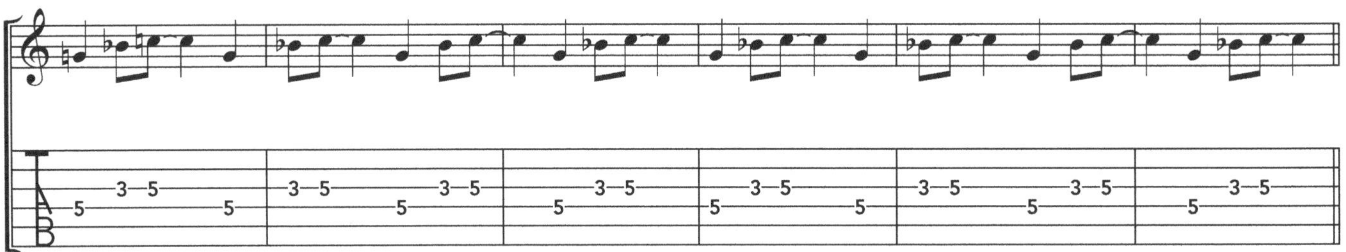

Example 20

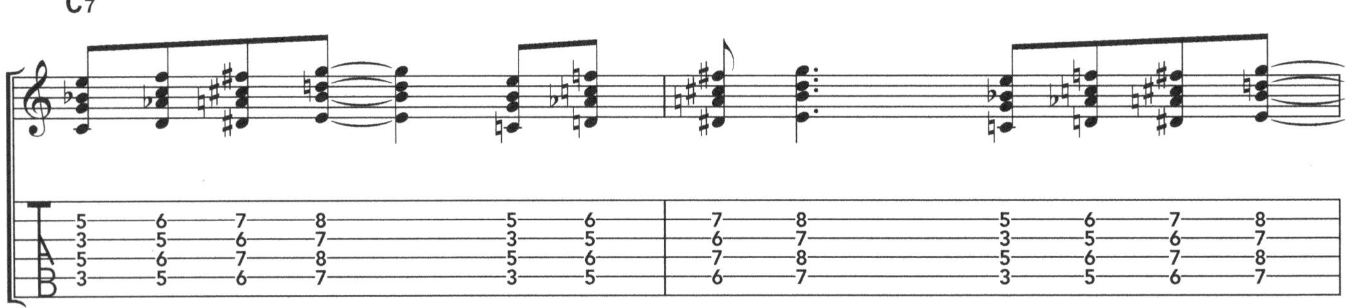

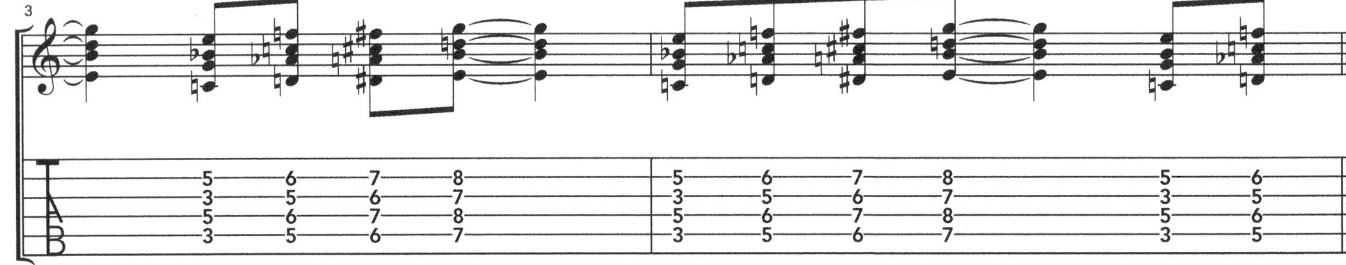

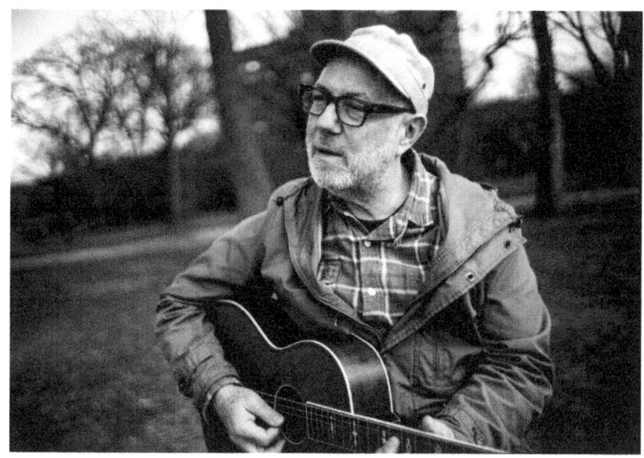

Adam Levy on Creative Practicing

Believe it or not, some players love practicing. They're stoked to fire up the metronome and work out on the strings daily, without any outside motivation. If you're one of those folks, you can skip this sidebar. If not, read on. I want to share three things that reliably get me into the right headspace on those days when all I can think of are the 37 other things I'd rather be doing.

Write something. Practicing and composing may seem to be very different activities, but writing is nearly always time well spent. Say, for example, you're trying to better understand altered-dominant sounds. Sure, you could work on some spicy chord voicings or their scalar relatives, but why not pen a 16-bar étude that implements these in a musical context? Then you'll have something to come back to and keep working on later—perhaps adding variations. You might even develop your étude into a complete tune to play on your own or with friends. And every time you play it, you'll have the opportunity to further explore altered-dominant sounds.

Practice the things that you really need to practice. Don't fall prey to trends on YouTube or other social media ("Five Diminished Arpeggio Forms You Must Know," for example). Such lessons may be useful, but just as often they're merely clickbait. Practice time is too precious for that! At the beginning of each month, write down three musical things that are most important to you. Then focus the majority of your practice time on activities that will help you improve in those specific areas.

Play along with records. Don't forget what it is we're practicing for: To make music. So, why not put on some music and play along? I don't mean copying parts that are already there—though that can be useful, too. What I'm proposing is that you play along as if you're in the band. Find a tone that complements what's already there and find a part (repetitive or freewheeling) that works.

—Adam Levy

Learning by Ear

Compared to, say, pianists or violinists, most guitarists didn't necessarily grow up reading music. Many learned to play songs by ear after listening to records over and over, developing strong aural skills compared to other instrumentalists. Nothing can replace the sweat equity of listening to the same lick a hundred times, trying repeatedly to capture the notes, tone, and time-feel. Those experiences—as challenging as they can be—often shape your ability to hear and remember quite a bit of music, which will serve you well on the bandstand and when playing with other musicians.

These days, it's easy to look online for tabs or quick lessons, but it's always better to trust your own ears. (I've seen many online tabs and lessons that were flat-out wrong, and I warn my own students about this.) Like anything, playing by ear takes a lot of patience and practice, but here are a few tips to get you going.

- If you don't already know it well, listen to the song repeatedly so that you can sing along with the essential parts of the melody, chord progression, or solo you're learning.
- When learning chord progressions, listen to and learn the bass note first, and try to identify whether the bass is playing the root of the chord or something else.
- When learning chord voicings, try to pick out the top note first, followed by the lowest note in the chord. Try to hear the tonality: is it major, minor, dominant, or something else? Then try to establish the register, string placement, or anything special such as the texture of open strings, an alternate tuning, harmonics, etc. Can you tell how many notes are in the voicing? If you can identify the lowest and highest note, plus the character of the chord, usually it's a matter of filling in the other notes based on what chord it is.
- If you're learning a fast solo line, try to split up the line by the beat and focus on the first note of each beat. For example, if it's a long, fast 16th-note line over the span of a full measure, try to determine the first 16th note of each beat. What is the arc of the line? Does it go up or down? Does it sound like a scale, an arpeggio, or something chromatic with a lot of half-steps? Identify the type of chord and then the sound of the chord scale. Let's say it's a fast, descending line over Cm7; you can identify the first notes of each beat and recognize the sound of C Dorian C D E♭ F G A B♭). Then it's just a matter of using your knowledge of theory to fill in the rest of the notes and find a good fingering that will enable you to play it at tempo.
- Try to ascertain tonal attributes of the guitar. Start with a macro analysis: Is it a steel-string or nylon? Maybe a 12-string? Maybe a resonator guitar? Is it a Telecaster or Stratocaster, or maybe a hollowbody? What kind of effects are being used? If it's an acoustic, any idea on miking techniques? Spending some time on aural analysis will sharpen your ears and fine-tune your awareness of the music happening around you the next time you perform.

CHAPTER EIGHT

Creative Practicing
Part Two

"You can't use up creativity. The more you use, the more you have."
–MAYA ANGELOU

In the last chapter, we explored the different stages and types of practice that can be beneficial throughout your trajectory and growth. If nothing else, we can agree that there is no one way to practice, but rather a variety of approaches that will all contribute to your development.

Consistent practice is certainly a key to success, but it's important to recognize there are other ways to practice creatively—even if you must go a few days without playing the guitar. In this chapter, we'll continue our exploration by looking at some common elements of a successful practice session, tips on learning new music, and the benefits of active listening and personal analysis. Finally, we'll look at a few different sample routines that you can apply to your own objectives and time availability.

Prelude No. 8

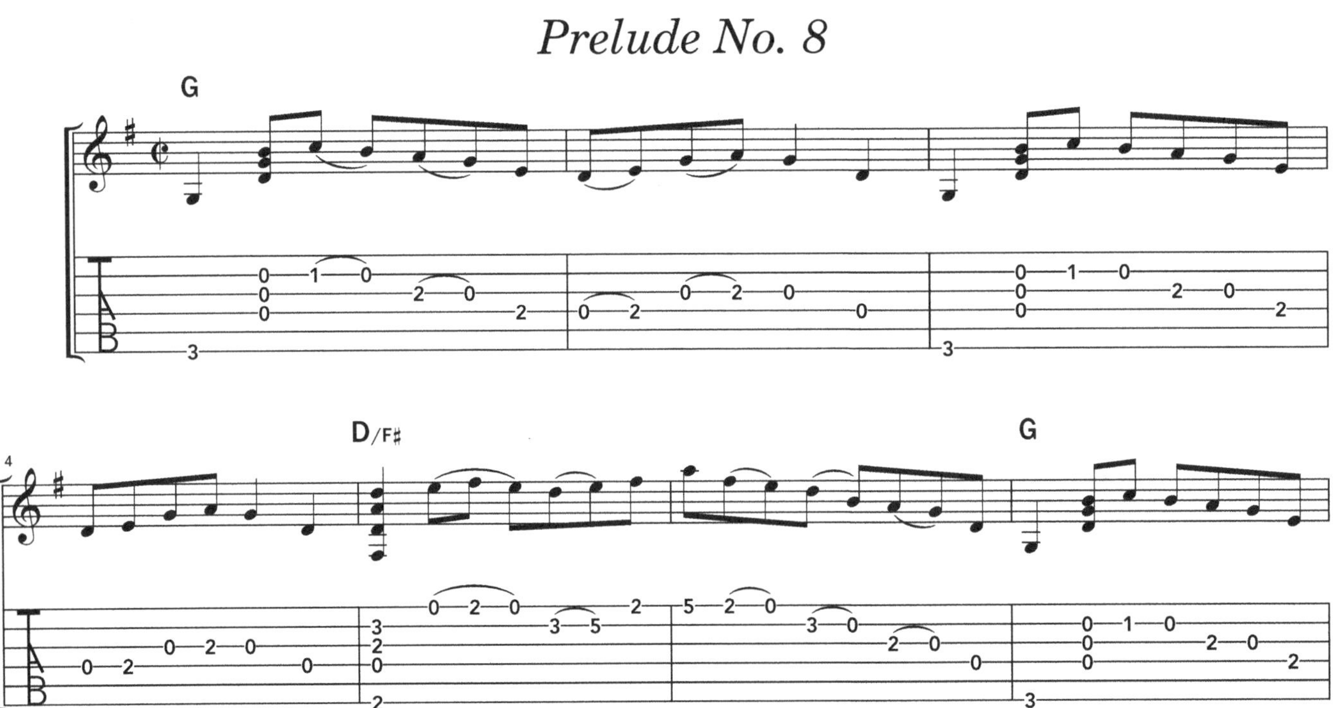

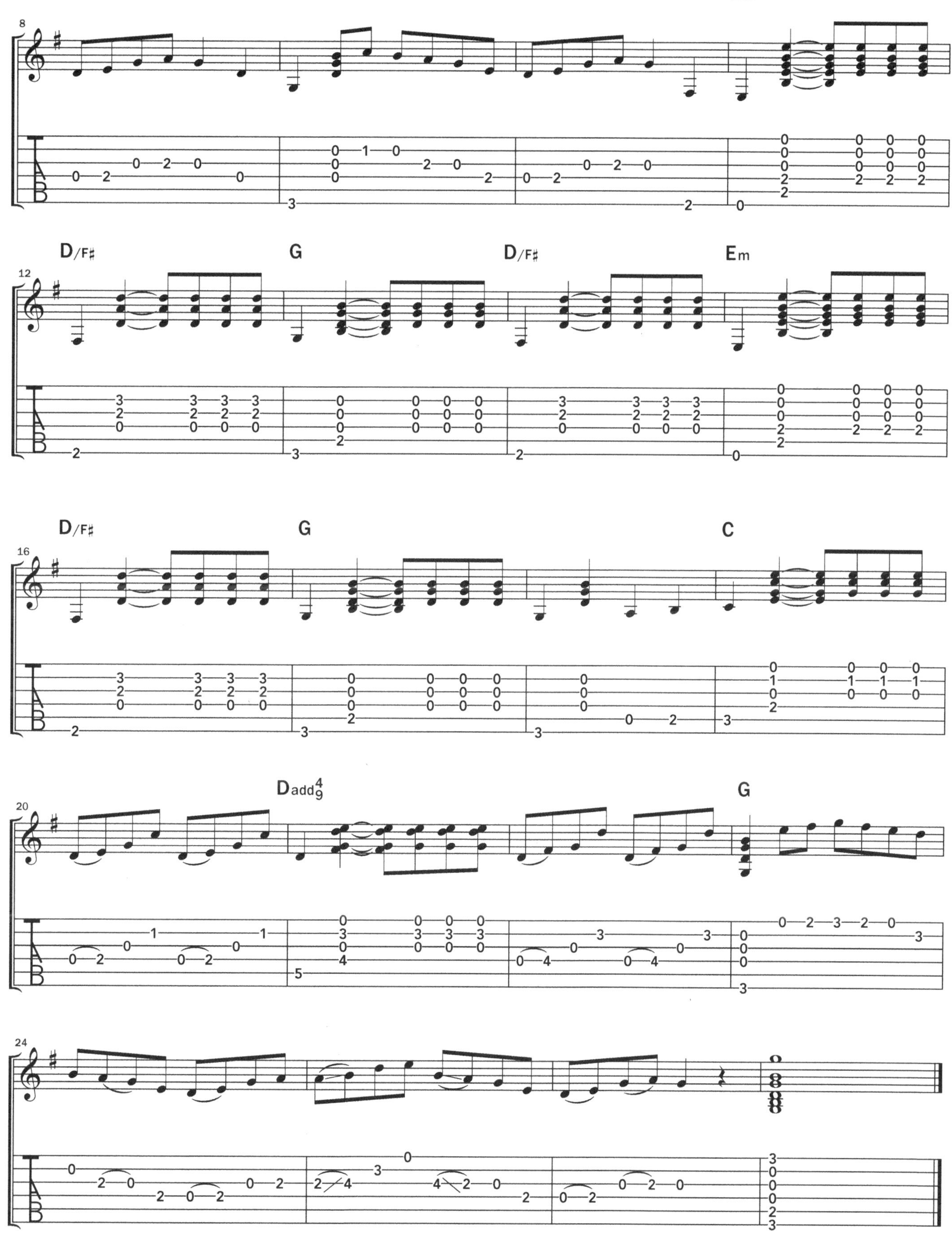

Em
D/F♯
G
D/F♯
Em
D/F♯
G
C
Dadd4/9
G

Elements of a Good Practice Session

Practice sessions are often dictated by how much time you may have, as well as by inspiration, motivation, requirements such as an upcoming concert, and general interest. In my view, there really isn't such a thing as the perfect practice routine, though it should include a basic warm-up before and cool-down afterward—and it should always be enjoyable. But here's a brief list of different types of practice that may be worth considering as you establish your own different routines, which could include:

1. Professional practice (learning music and/or technical skills specifically related to an upcoming gig or tour)
2. Casual practice (simply for the enjoyment of playing)
3. Maintenance (keeping the hands limber, the mind fresh, and the ears wide open)
4. Learning new concepts (transcribing, working out of a book, taking lessons, creating your own techniques, etc.)
5. Listening (while some musicians don't necessarily consider listening to be practice, in-depth, analytical listening is one of the best ways to practice and improve)
6. Tone production (working on your tone and your personal approach, recording yourself and listening back, etc.)
7. Music fundamentals (sight-reading, fretboard exercises, scales, arpeggios, chord voicings and voice-leading, basic rhythm and technical exercises)

Try not to force a practice session if you're too busy or distracted emotionally or physically. It's better to take the day off, or even a few if need be. Don't worry—your talent and years of hard work won't disappear after a few days. Sometimes, though, practicing and playing music when you don't feel like it or when you're going through something is just the right thing to make you feel better. There have been many times that I've had a gig when I didn't feel well, was exhausted, or upset about something in my life. Once I began playing, I felt much better—healed, in fact. In my view, this is just one example of the many healing properties of music.

When you are busy with the demands of personal and professional life—this is common for touring musicians, for instance—you can combine a limited practice session that focuses on maintenance (e.g., technical exercises and repertoire) with visualization (practicing in your mind and active listening).

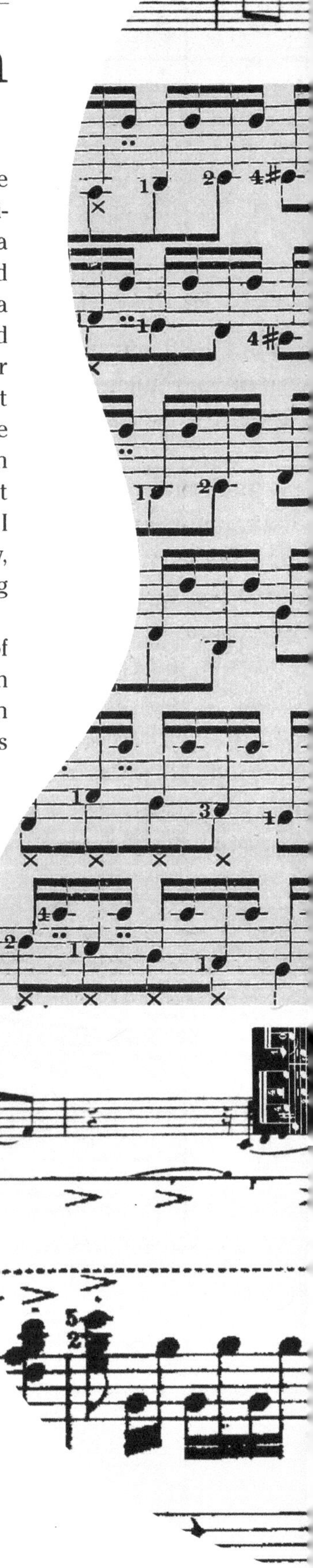

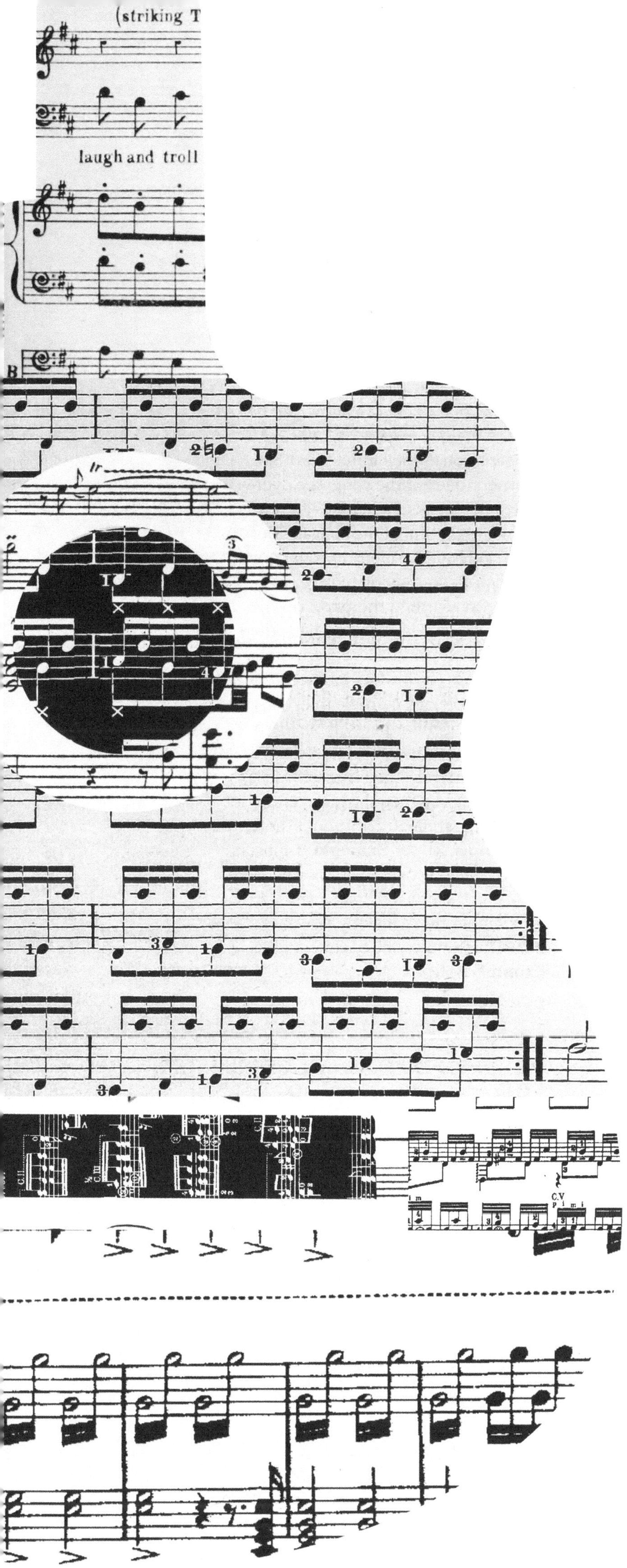

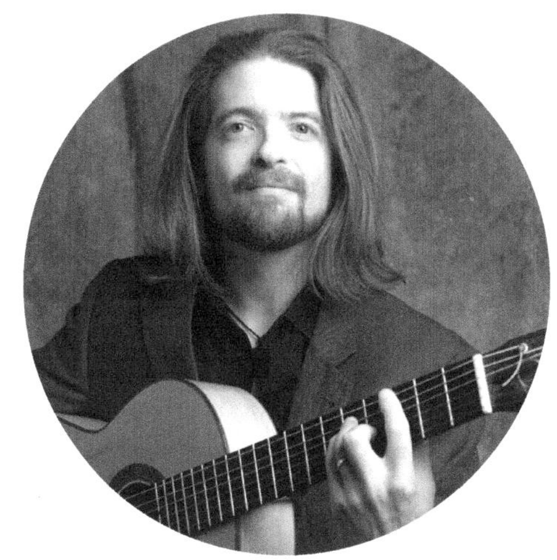

Juanito Pascual
For Flamenco Guitarists

Flamenco, which can present challenges that are different (or at least more apparent) than in other genres, requires a physically and technically demanding technique, as well as an understanding of a complex musical language and cultural traditions. After over 35 years of learning and playing flamenco, I've realized that many guitarists don't necessarily understand how to break things down, and therefore, they waste time with ineffective practice and/or injure themselves trying to achieve technical proficiency.

One solution applicable to any genre is dividing your study into three separate categories: rhythm, technique, and listening. This is most easily achieved by:

1. Allotting time to working with the rhythms away from your guitar by clapping along to recordings or rhythm tracks
2. Isolating the individual techniques (picado, arpeggio, rasgueado, alzapua, etc.) to develop comfort, good tone, and consistency
3. Listening to and watching a lot of flamenco daily to assimilate the core essence and nuances of the style

In other words, many people try to play flamenco without a firm grasp of these elements, and they struggle to play because they do not have a clear sense of *how it should sound*. This is common among students of flamenco, and separating these three elements, beginning with listening, can greatly improve your ability to play a new style and save considerable time and frustration.

—Juanito Pascual

Learning New Music

Learning new music to add to your repertoire, for study, or just for sheer enjoyment can be one of the most rewarding aspects of practice. I've found that learning starts with listening, which is often most effective away from the guitar to avoid any distractions. Find a quiet environment that allows for deep, uninterrupted listening through a quality set of headphones or speakers.

If you're learning a song that has been recorded numerous times, find the original version first. Listen to it two or three times just to get the sound into your ears. Then you can start analyzing (again, even before you pick up the guitar) by writing your observations down. Begin by answering the following questions: What is the overall form of the song? What are the time and key signatures? Does it sound like it's in a major or minor tonality? Or maybe something else, like a static modal piece or a song that explores multiple tonalities and key centers? Does it modulate clearly? Do the chords seem relatively simple or complex? What is the tempo or general feel? Can you describe it with a genre or historic time period? How many measures are in each section? Can you determine the chord progression without using your guitar?

The more you can home in on these details before trying to play the song, the easier learning it on the guitar will be, and the deeper you will learn it; in other words, the less likely you are to forget it. Learn the melody by ear—or by following along with sheet music if you have it—and then sing along until you have memorized it for the most part. Again, this will allow you to connect with the melody organically, not by a memorized fingering on the guitar fretboard. Sing along with cornerstones of the song, the overall groove, rhythmic breaks, repeating riffs, etc. Feel the groove and rhythm of the song in your body and the melody and harmony in your ears.

Once you pick up your guitar, you're ready to dive in! I suggest learning the parts on the guitar in the following order: melody first; the root notes of each chord in the progression; the full chord voicings (trying to capture extensions, open-string voicings if applicable, etc.); followed by the actual guitar parts. If I'm learning something like a jazz or pop standard, I'll play through several times starting with just the melody (**Example 1**), then the basic chord progression, adding some substitutions here and there (**Example 2**). As **Example 3** illustrates, playing the melody over the bass creates a nice counterpoint exercise. Finally, you can put together a simple chord melody, which will give you a basic arrangement of the song as shown in **Example 4**.

Example 1

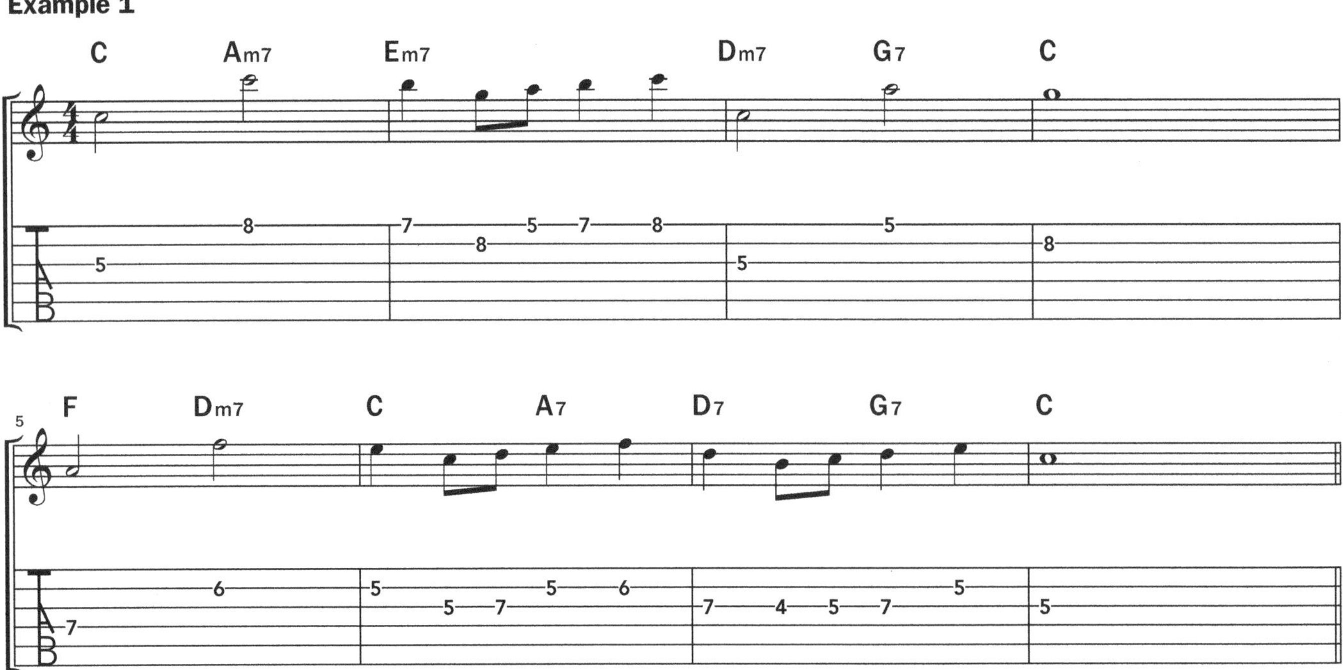

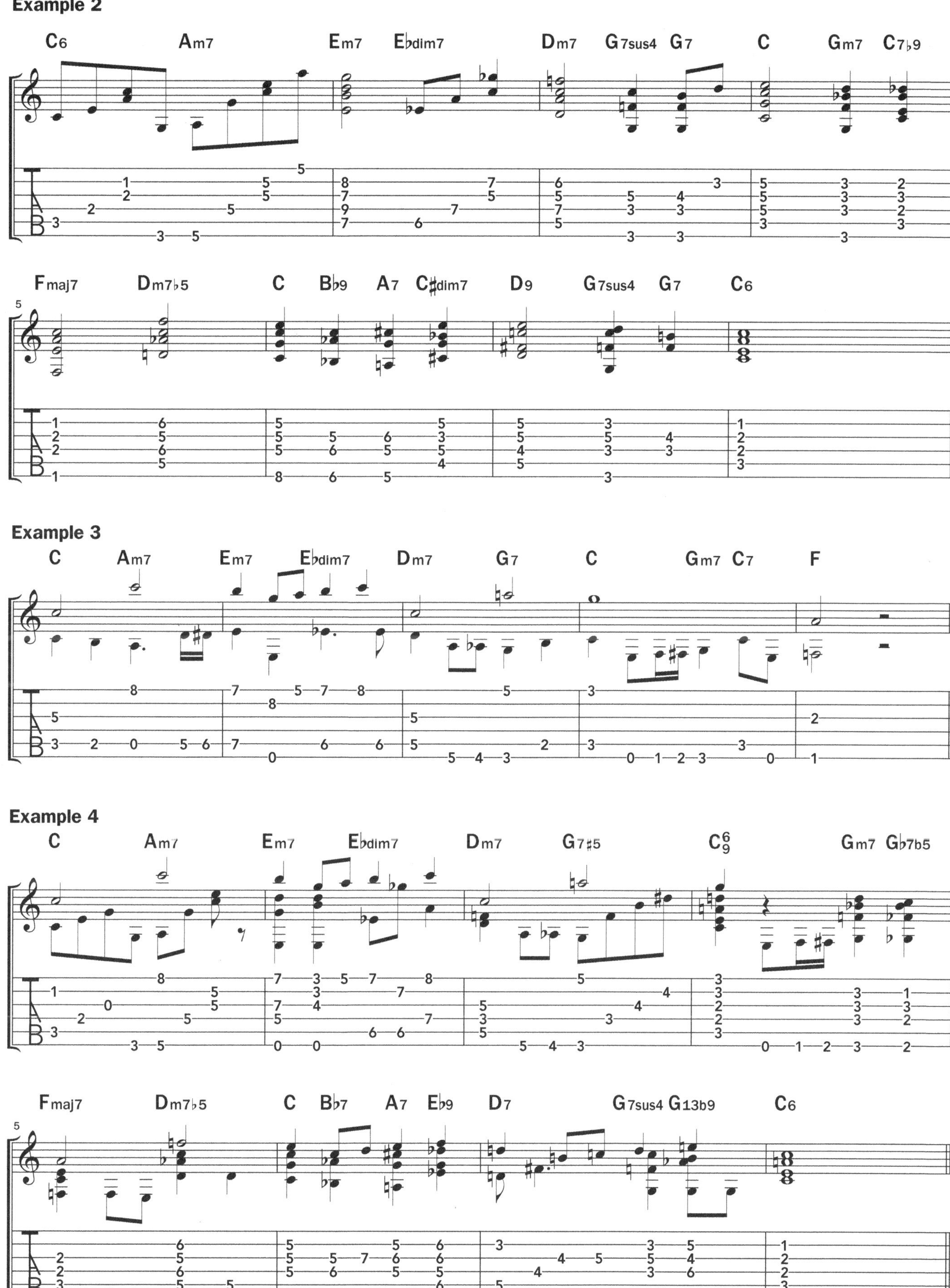
Example 2
C6 Am7 Em7 E♭dim7 Dm7 G7sus4 G7 C Gm7 C7♭9
5
Fmaj7 Dm7♭5 C B♭9 A7 C♯dim7 D9 G7sus4 G7 C6
Example 3
C Am7 Em7 E♭dim7 Dm7 G7 C Gm7 C7 F
Example 4
C Am7 Em7 E♭dim7 Dm7 G7♯5 C6/9 Gm7 G♭7b5
5
Fmaj7 Dm7♭5 C B♭7 A7 E♭9 D7 G7sus4 G13b9 C6

The next steps might be to practice and/or arrange the melody within the context of a solo piece or playing parts with a band. After learning the melody, try practicing it by playing it in different fretboard locations and string sets (**Example 5**). You could play it in octaves (**Example 6**) or add embellishments to the basic melody (**Example 7**). Another way is to create some interesting counterpoint by adding a simple harmony part to the melody, as shown in **Example 8**.

If you are studying the song to add to your long-term repertoire, you could practice ways to reinforce your knowledge of the song, and music theory in general. For instance, once you've memorized the chord progression, play it in a different key. **Example 9** transposes our melody in the key of C to the key of A major.

Jazz guitarist Joe Pass was well known for his ability to play a song in any key, and he often modulated through several different keys when he played a 12-bar blues. A great place to start is by understanding the diatonic chords of any major key identified by Roman numerals, uppercase for major and lowercase for minor chord qualities, and writing out and playing in different keys (**Examples 10** and **11**).

This is also the basis of the Nashville number system, which really helps to identify chord progressions by scale degree and interval movements. Try using the numbers to easily transpose from one key to another (**Examples 12** and **13**). You could also transcribe chord voicings, solos, breaks, or the entire arrangement from a recorded version you like. All of these are invaluable activities that will bring you closer to understanding the innate details of music.

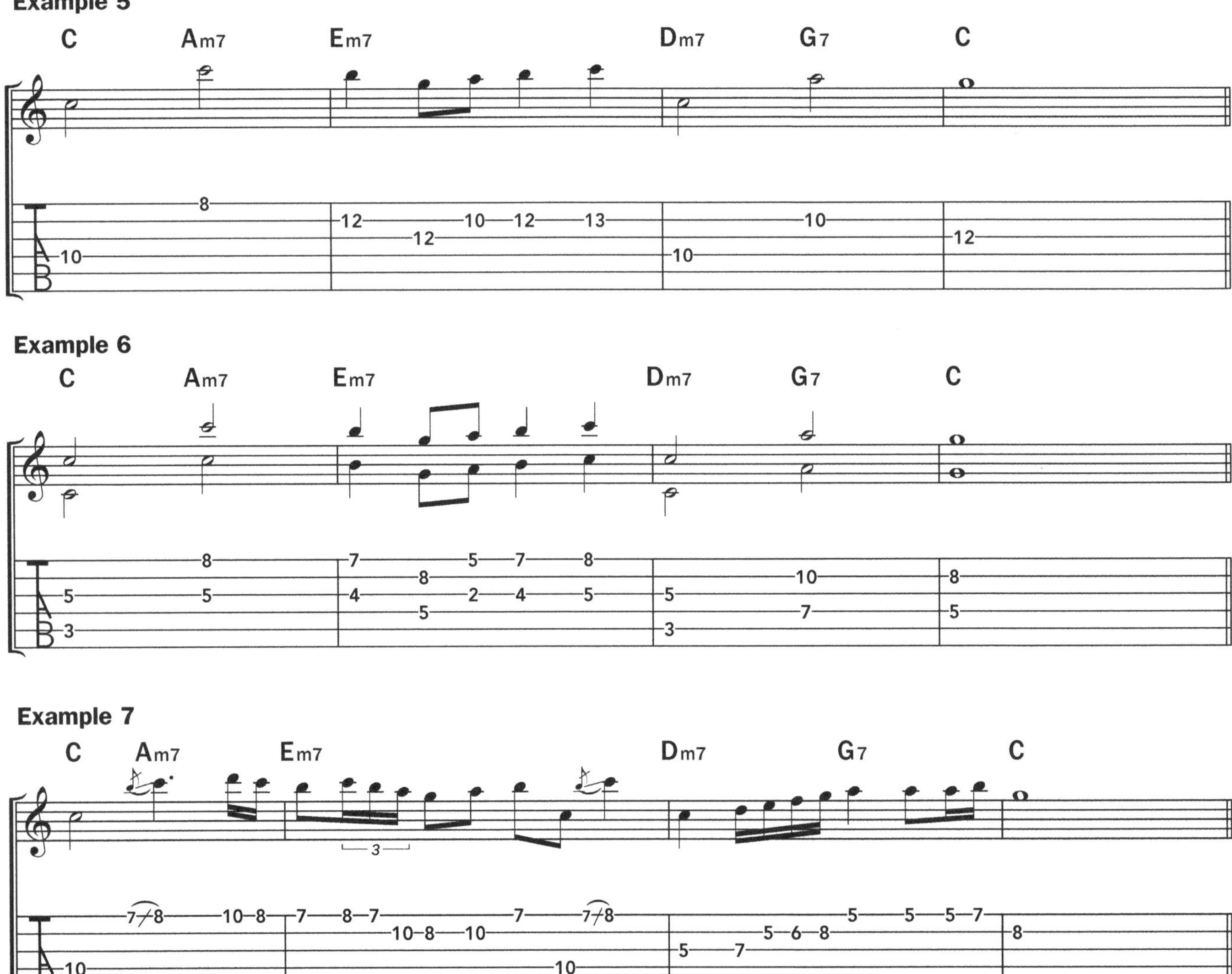

Example 8

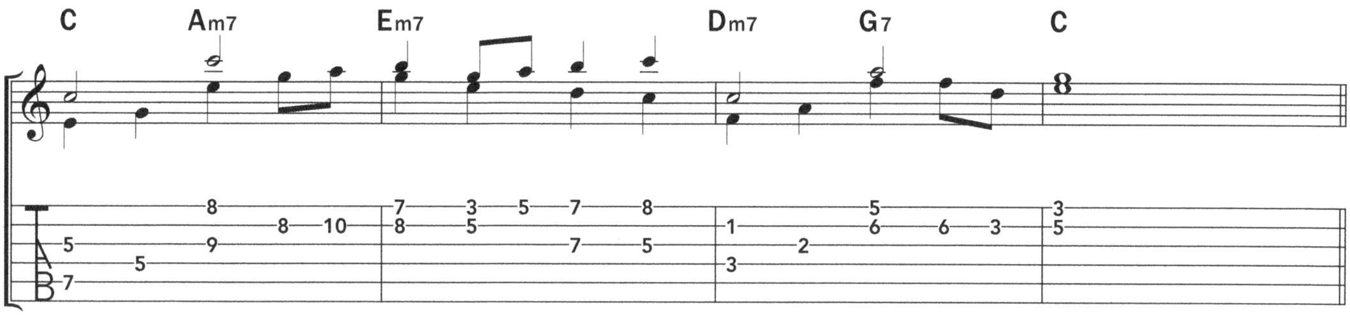

C
Am7
Em7
Dm7
G7
C

Example 9

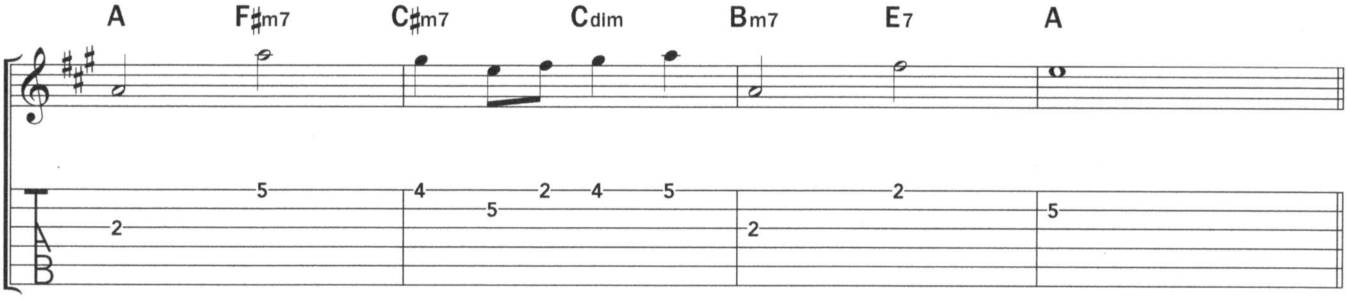

A
F♯m7
C♯m7
Cdim
Bm7
E7
A

Example 10

Example 11

Cmaj7 Dm7 Em7 Fmaj7
G7 Am7 Bm7♭5 Cmaj7
Amaj7 Bm7 C♯m7 Dmaj7
E7 F♯m7 G♯m7♭5 Amaj7

Example 12

Cmaj7
Am7
Em7
E♭dim7
Dm7
G7
Cmaj7

Example 13

Amaj7
F♯m7
C♯m7
Cdim7
Bm7
E7
Amaj7

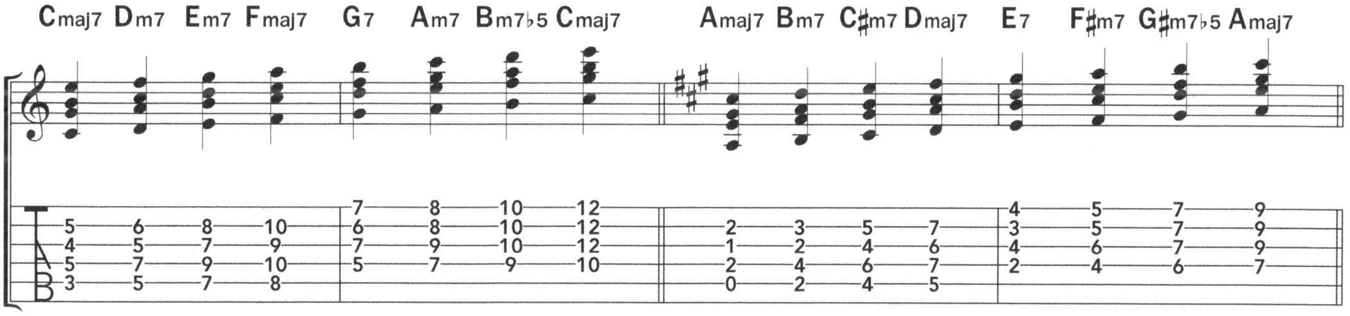

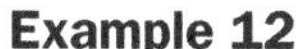

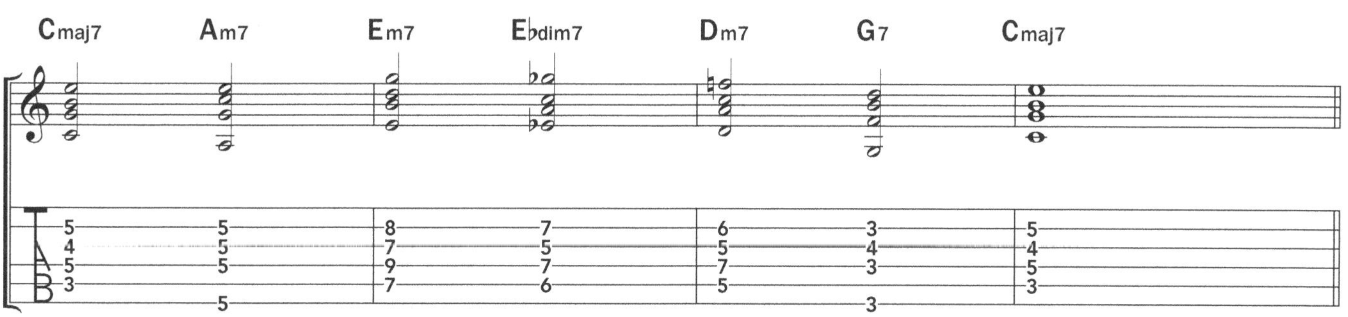

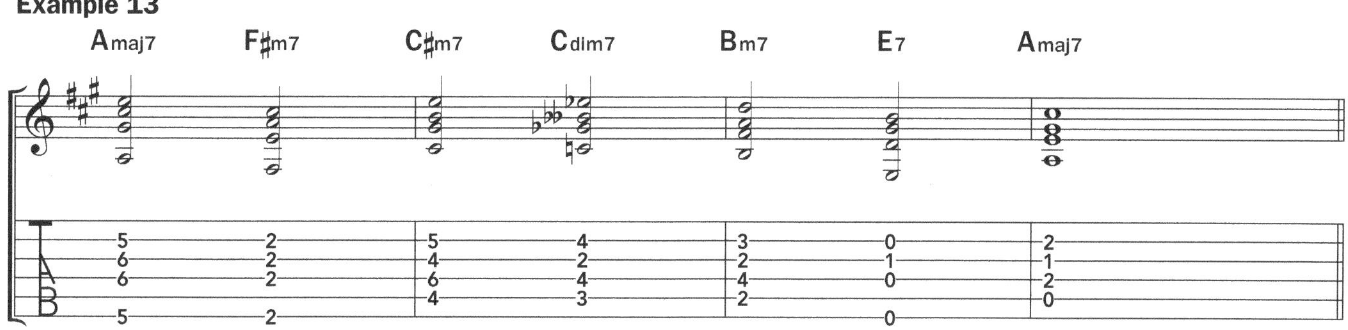

Active Listening as Practice

In my years as an educator, I have often been surprised by students who want to play a particular style of music—jazz, for example—but never actually listen to it or study its history and players. Students of jazz guitar simply cannot internalize the language and deep traditions of the music without listening to it regularly (obsessively, even!) and relying solely on *The Real Book* to learn and play songs.

While fakebooks (i.e., songbooks) and play-along apps can serve as great learning aids and practice tools, they cannot replace the deep sensory experience of intensive listening and ultimately playing with other musicians in that style. Nor can these tools replace the profound joy of learning something new and the accompanying gift and satisfaction of a new means of expression. Indeed, the tradition of learning jazz guitar—as with so many other styles and traditions—is based on the aural experiences of listening to music on the radio, recordings, and live performances.

Jazz guitarist Tal Farlow once reflected on this modality of learning music and training his ears: "I used to listen to all those broadcasts of the big bands coming over the radio... since I listened to the radio so much, I knew all the popular tunes of the day. So, when I played with local bands, I already knew most of the tunes. If I didn't know the tune, then I would use my ear to match up with what I heard the band doing."

Wes Montgomery, who stated that he once learned Charlie Christian's solos to play on the bandstand before he developed his own style, declared, "Sometimes I'll do nothing but listen to records. All kinds—over and over." The simple act of repetition can be a powerful way of internalizing vocabulary, whether it's listening to one song or recording over and over or playing a line or complete solo repeatedly for days or even weeks.

However, at times it can be important to balance active and intense listening with a period of not listening to anything and instead focusing on the sound in your imagination. A follow-up quote from Montgomery: "Then after a while, it breaks, and I don't even want to hear (records). Nothing. I think it's because at the times I don't want to hear, I've heard so much it's got me confused and I'm so far away from it on my instrument—from the things I've been hearing—that I've got to put it aside and go back to where I am. And try to get out of that hole!"

This last statement is a testament to how it can sometimes feel discouraging listening to a lot of music that may seem beyond your abilities at the time. This is normal, and at these moments, it may be helpful to take a break from listening to your favorite music. Vocalist Bobby McFerrin recalled that he once spent a period of several months not listening to any music, and simply devoting his time to singing and developing his unique vocal style.

Sample Practice Routines

Regardless of how much time you have for practice, a good rule of thumb is to try to have a clear plan in place and create an arc to your session. Something that looks like the following:

- Warming up the hands and body with stretching: 5 minutes
- Quick guitar warm-up: 5 minutes
- Something easy and fun to play, e.g. a song or étude you know well, or a simple groove: 5 minutes
- Topic or concept: 30 minutes
- Break: 5 minutes, or, if ending for the day, finish with a cool-down/free-form improv

A guitar warm-up could consist of simple chord voicings that involve finger coordination (**Examples 14** and **15**), basic scales (**Example 16**), or arpeggio patterns (**Example 17**). The main difference between a warm-up and a technical workout is the duration and intensity. In the warm-up, the goal is to wake up the hands and connect with the guitar, without fatiguing the hands or risking injury by playing something too strenuous or difficult while still cold.

A great way to conclude any session is with a cool-down or improvisation. A cool-down might involve playing a basic riff or reviewing a new technique. Improvising is also an excellent way to review and conclude a session. This could involve playing along to a backing track, improvising single-note lines or chord forms, or engaging in total free-form playing, letting whatever comes to mind flow naturally.

This basic outline of a routine will keep your session around 45-50 minutes, after which you should take a break. Maybe stretch a bit, go for a short walk, or drink water—something that allows your practice work to sink in and gives your body a short rest. If you want or need to practice longer than 45 minutes to an hour, make sure to break up those sessions into different times of the day if possible. Otherwise, strive for a cadence of 35-45 minutes of practice followed by a 15-minute break, then practice, break, etc.

Turn to page 122 for three sample routines based on the duration of your practice session and your goals—whether preparing for a series of performances, learning, or general maintenance when you're short on time.

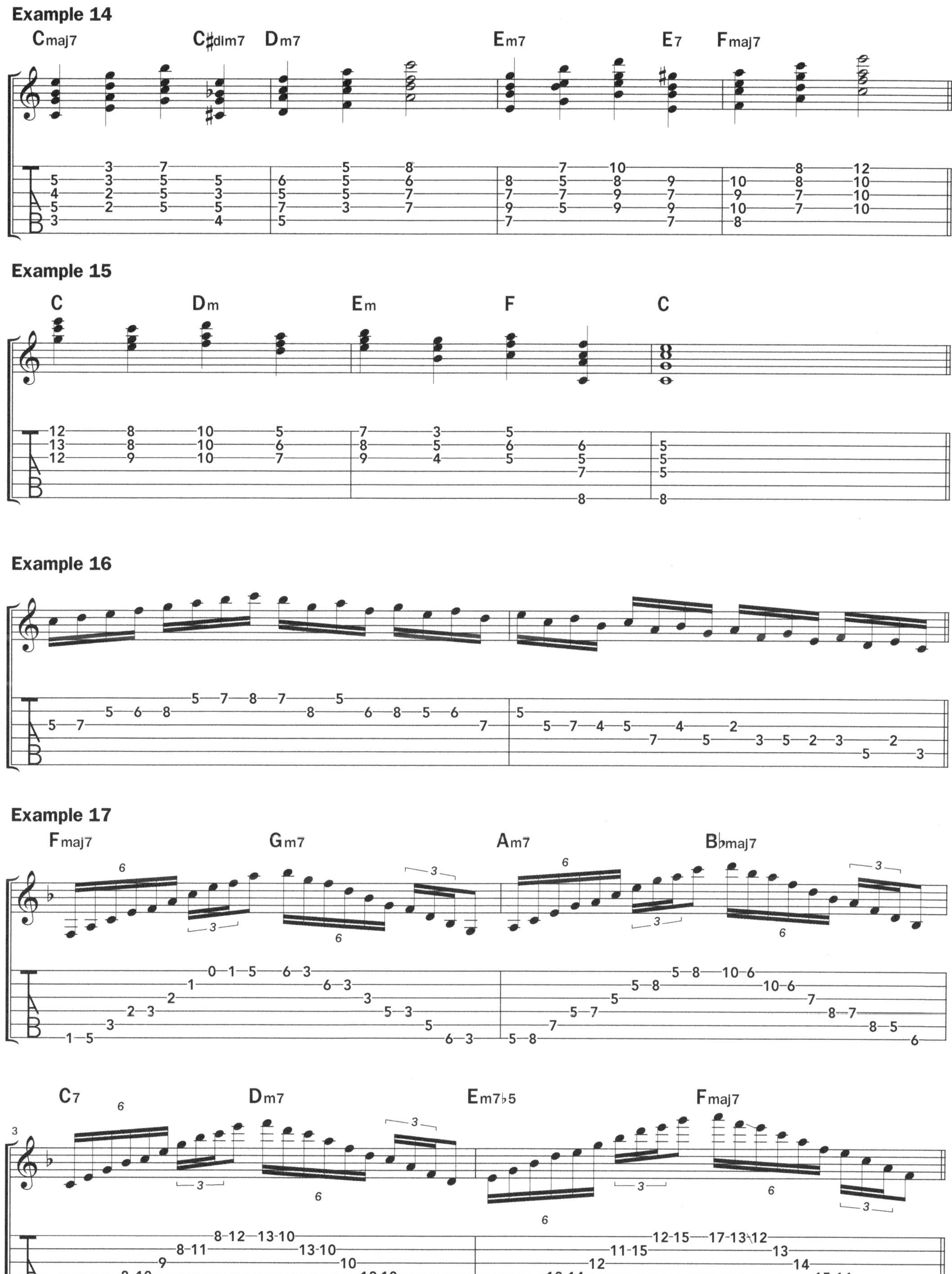
Example 14
Cmaj7 C♯dim7 Dm7 Em7 E7 Fmaj7
Example 15
C Dm Em F C
Example 16
Example 17
Fmaj7 Gm7 Am7 B♭maj7
C7 Dm7 Em7♭5 Fmaj7

Practice Routine #1

Preparing for a gig, performance series, tour (three to four hours)

- Physical stretching prior to the first session; mentally organizing your practice material; emptying the mind *(5–10 minutes)*
- Guitar warm-ups *(5–10 minutes)*
- Repertoire #1 *(40 minutes)*
- Break *(15 minutes)*
- Repertoire #2 *(40 minutes)*
- Break *(15 minutes)*
- Repertoire #3 *(40 minutes)*
- Break *(15 minutes)*
- Repertoire #4 *(40 minutes)*
- Cool-down/improv *(5–10 minutes)*

Depending on the type of performance, your practice time might involve different aspects of working on repertoire, which may include:

- Listening to the source music
- Learning the music through sheet music, recordings, charts, etc.
- Transcribing guitar parts
- Arranging original compositions
- Working on specific techniques for songs
- Working on tone production, sound and/or gear settings, special effects
- Planning for alternate tunings and sequence, if applicable
- Setting and practicing tempos for songs
- Determining set list and practicing transitions, stories about songs, etc.

This last aspect is an example of something musicians don't typically think of as practice material, but learning how to connect with an audience, stalling for extra time when necessary, tuning your guitar quickly and efficiently (or changing a string on stage if need be), and practicing physical and musical transitions between songs are all ingredients for a successful performance.

Another aspect to consider: If you are planning to practice for three-plus hours in a single day, break up the sessions, e.g., in two-hour chunks, whenever possible. For instance, you might spend two hours in the morning, take a longer break, and then return to practice later in the afternoon or evening. Begin every practice session by stretching your body and hands, plus some basic guitar warm-ups.

Practice Routine #2

Learning new concepts and/or general practice (two to three hours)

- Stretching *(5–10 minutes)*
- Guitar warm-ups *(5–10 minutes)*
- Topic #1 *(40 minutes)*
- Break *(15 minutes)*
- Topic #2 *(40 minutes)*
- Break *(15 minutes)*
- Musicianship *(40 minutes)*
- Cool-down/improv *(5–10 minutes)*

This routine resembles a session that a student might use, and the subjects or topics may vary based on what they wish to improve. These topics might include:

- Learning and memorizing new chord voicings
- Improvising over a chord progression
- Learning and practicing new techniques (picking, articulation, extended fretting, hybrid picking, fingerstyle, harmonics, percussive effects, strumming patterns, etc.)
- Learning and practicing a transcription of a guitar or other instrument solo
- Composing and/or arranging new music
- Repertoire practice

Obviously, there are many different topics to explore and work on, and this is where a practice journal can help you organize a lot of different material and track your progress. You might want to work on onc particular topic a couple of times a day for a week or more, or you may choose to work on several different topics over the course of a week. Don't worry about being too stringent, and give yourself flexibility when you need it.

Regarding musicianship as part of this routine, you could work on and alternate:

- Fretboard studies (note location, patterns, harmonic cycles)
- Rhythm and metronome practice
- Sight-reading standard music notation
- Ear-training (software training programs, play and sing, identify intervals and chords, transcribe songs and solos from recordings, etc.)
- General studies in harmony, form, music history, reading

When practice time is limited, it's always better to get a little time in rather than no time at all. When practicing for maintenance, focus on fundamentals such as technical exercises (scales, arpeggios, rudiments, patterns, études), repertoire (excerpts of several songs or a work in progress), and taking time to connect with your instrument through improvisation (taking a solo or improvising rhythm parts or chord progressions).

Practice Routine #3

Maintenance and/or limited time to play (20–45 minutes)

- Stretching *(5 minutes)*
- Guitar warm-ups *(2 minutes)*
- Practice material—fundamentals, technique, limited repertoire *(10–30 minutes)*
- Cool-down/improv *(3–5 minutes)*

CHAPTER NINE

Good Medicine

Advice for the Long Haul

"I never practice my guitar... from time to time I just open the case and throw in a piece of raw meat."

—WES MONTGOMERY

As guitarists, we want to play the music we love, pain- and injury-free, for the rest of our lives. We are in this for the long haul. That's an incredible endeavor, and a gift! One can easily devote an entire lifetime to the study of music and the enjoyment of playing guitar. We have all experienced the palpable benefits—physical, mental, emotional, and spiritual—of playing the guitar and music, with friends or simply alone with our instrument.

While writing this book, I reached out to good friends, colleagues, and guitar heroes of mine to share their experiences, perspectives, and advice on a number of topics ranging from staying healthy to practicing to staying creative and inspired. Following are responses by acclaimed guitarists Clive Carroll, Alex de Grassi, Eric Johnson, Laurence Juber, Vicki Genfan, Grant Gordy, and Juanito Pascual pertaining to each topic in no particular order. I like to think of their responses as good medicine. They have all dedicated their lives to creating the best version of themselves through their music, practice, and dedication to the guitar, and we are all the better for it, receiving their gifts through recordings and live performances.

Prelude No. 9

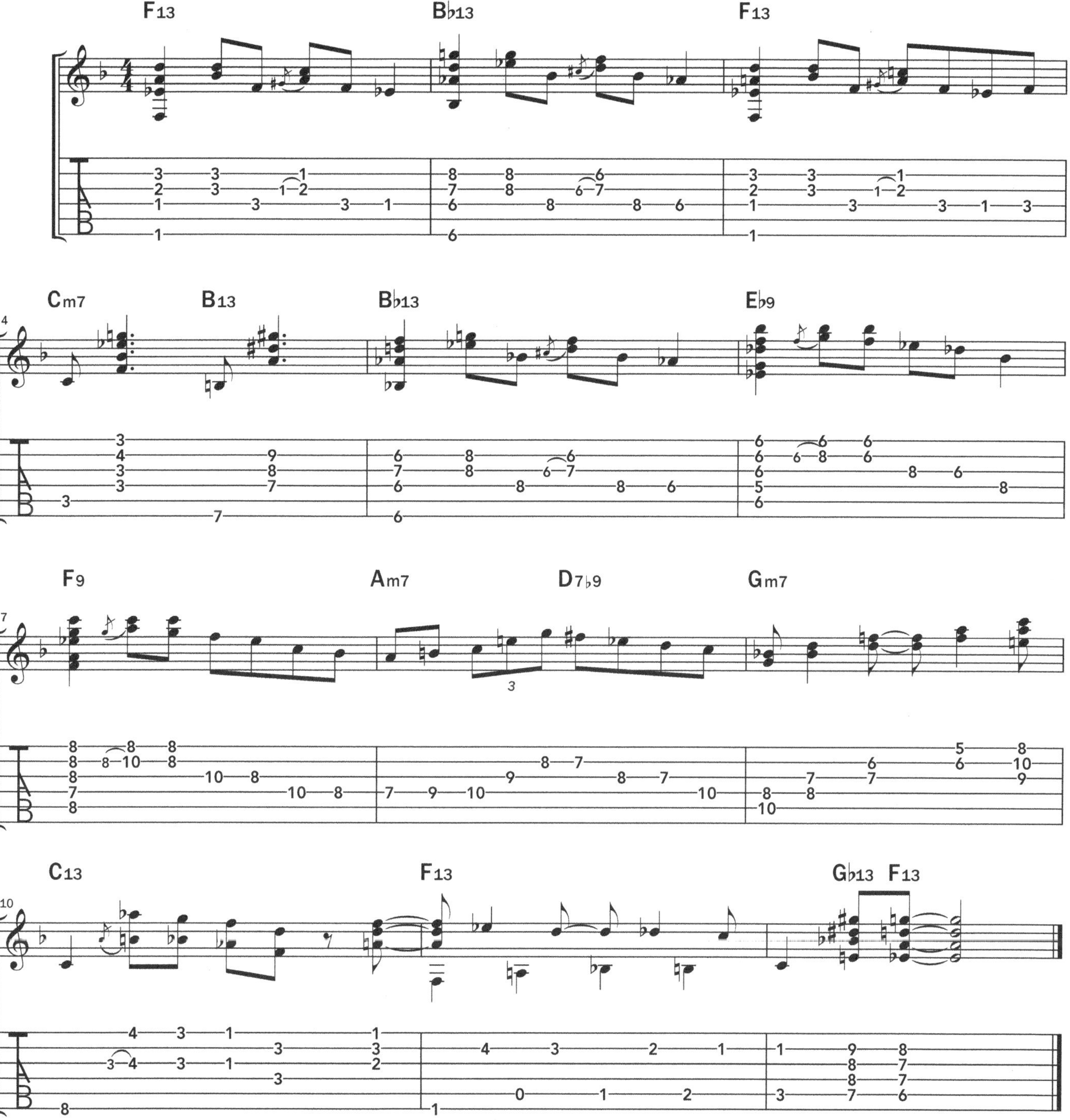

On Practicing

Guitarists often have a hard time identifying what exactly to practice. Whether it's because they feel they don't have much time and aren't sure what to prioritize, or maybe they have so much they want to work on, they're not quite sure where or how to start, and ultimately, they get discouraged. Eric Johnson lets his intuition guide his practice sessions. "Something interesting I find is that if I sit down to practice and I observe the intuitive information that's coming from within me—rather than just letting my mind initiate the same musical phrases I repeat over and over—I become a listener. Intuition can, many times, open new doorways. It can also connect us with the mystical joy of tapping into the unexplainable magic of music."

Alex de Grassi also pays attention to intuition through improvisation informed by his knowledge of music theory. "I like to warm up with a bit of improv, maybe on a theme I've heard somewhere—traditional folk songs are a great resource—or even from one of my own compositions," de Grassi says. "I try playing the theme using different rhythms and/or time signatures, scales, cross-string scales, and all the articulations and different sonics that make the acoustic guitar such a versatile instrument. Plus," he continues, "a little theory is helpful. Understanding the Roman numeral system of chord progressions and modes is useful [if one wants] to change keys quickly.

Tone, dynamics, and articulations should not be overlooked; their color and depth that brings music alive—I love the 3D quality those elements bring to music!"

In addition to fundamentals such as harmony, voice-leading, and a keen awareness of style, Laurence Juber often emphasizes repertoire in his practice. Juber also works to keep things fresh: "I change up the environment, finding a different spot to play, exploring different keys, and being in the musical moment. Always listen and visualize the story you are telling with your music."

Grant Gordy will typically dedicate his practice time to fundamentals, especially ear training: "Learn how to hear better. The number one thing in music is listening. Make sure you can hear what you're doing—for example, be able to hear/sing/play the root, third, and fifth of any chord progression, and learn how to hear every other note in relation to the triad. Also focus on rhythm, groove, feel, tone, and functional harmony. Work on those things, and it will cover a lot of the bases!"

Developing a solid time-feel and rhythmic freedom is a high priority, too. "Practice with the metronome. Use it in challenging ways to test your ability to hear where beat 1 is. When you hear a tricky rhythmic phrase and you're not sure what's going on, sit with it and slowly digest it. Don't let it go until you can hear it and feel it. Listen to drummers!"

Clive Carroll also focuses on rhythmic training in his practice. "Rhythm and timing, no question. While a metronomic performance is, for the most part, non-musical, slow practice with one is extremely beneficial. If I'm performing a groove-based piece in front of an audience and the front row aren't tapping their feet, it's my fault, not theirs."

Carroll also integrates composition into his practice to stay fresh. "I find that the best way to practice in a creative way is through writing and/or arranging music. It expands my understanding of melodic and harmonic fretboard possibilities, rhythmic ideas that are exciting for the picking hand to try, and the finger independence gained from this path of study helps to pick out more detail in the pieces I think I already know!"

When asked about integrating creativity into a practice session, Gordy answers, "There are endless ways! Learn a solo from an instrument you don't play. Play metronome games. Take lessons from other musicians. Take a tune you know and learn it in a different key, or all twelve. See if you can write a tune in 30 minutes. It never ends or gets old."

He has also learned to let his body and mind tell him how to stay focused and when to stop: "Make sure to take breaks. Recently, I found that I could sustain intense focus on a hard piece for about 40 minutes before I started to feel myself lagging. Don't get distracted by the internet. You'll get a lot more out of practice time if that time isn't spent scrolling on your phone."

Juanito Pascual shares this philosophy with students and in his own practice: "Use a timer to build breaks into your practice. I recommend a maximum of 45 minutes at a time, followed by 10- to 15-minute breaks where you stand up and stretch a bit. For optimal physical function and mental clarity, I also recommend no more than three of these in a row. If I want to practice more than three hours per day, I try to break it up into two (if not three) different parts of the day."

Vicki Genfan

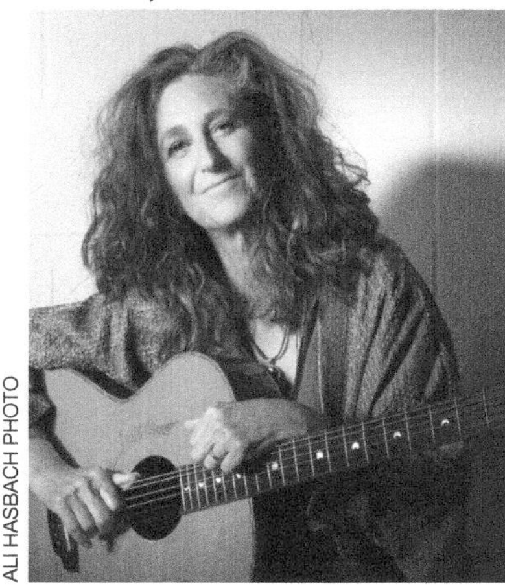

ALI HASBACH PHOTO

Grant Gordy

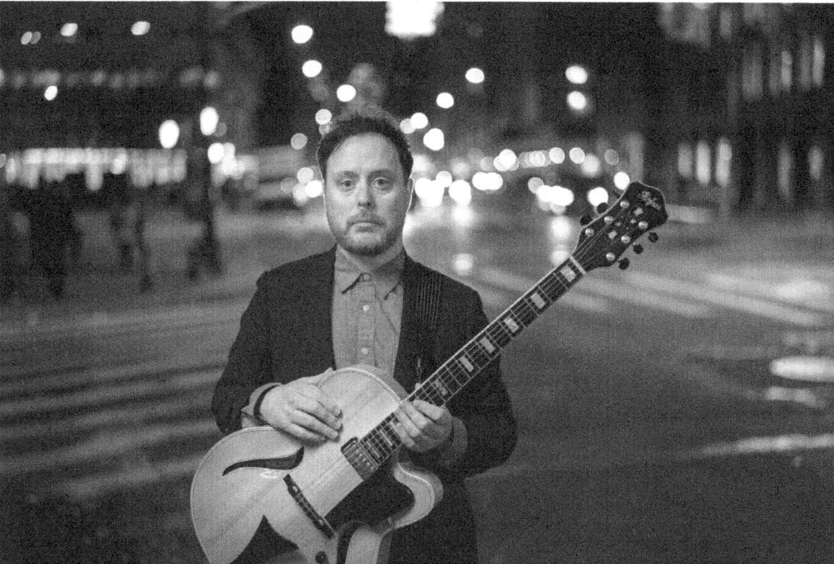

JOHN ROGERS PHOTO

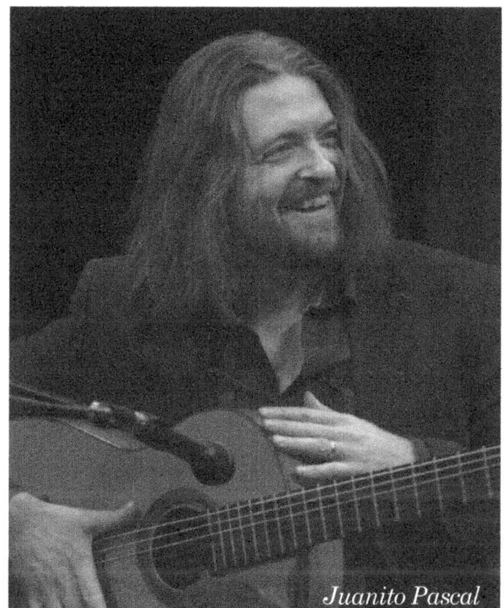

Juanito Pascal

ROCCO S. COVIELLO

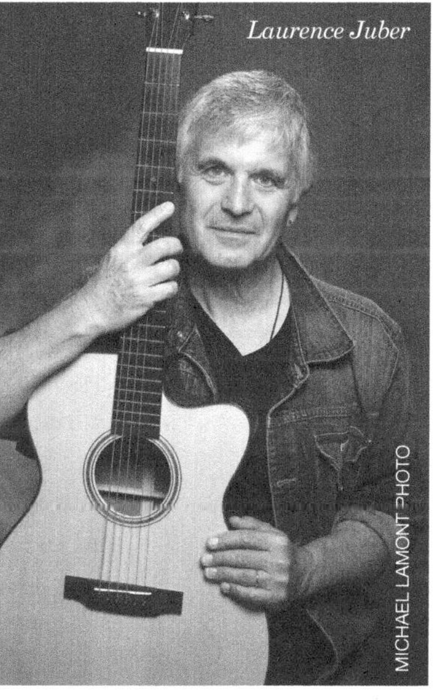

Laurence Juber

MICHAEL LAMONT PHOTO

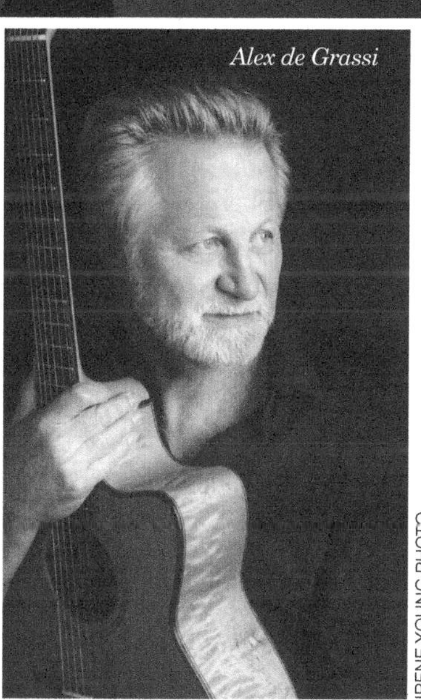

Alex de Grassi

IRENE YOUNG PHOTO

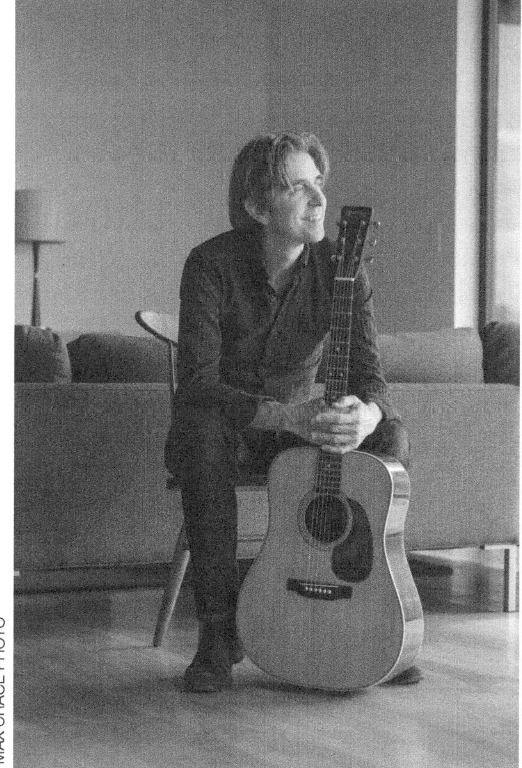

MAX CRACE PHOTO

Eric Johnson

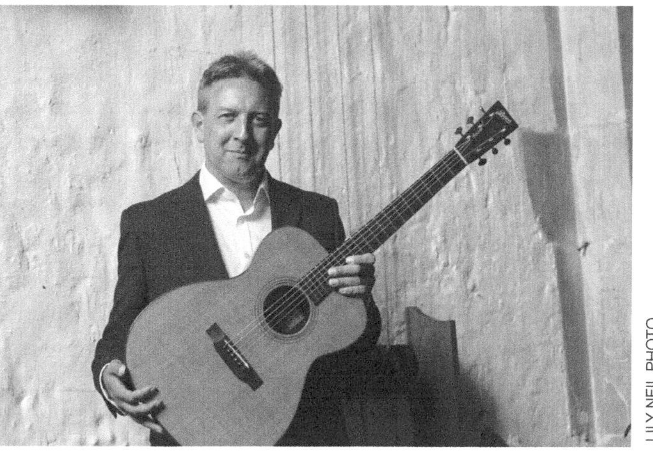

LILY NEIL PHOTO

Clive Carroll

On Technique

As just about every accomplished guitarist will attest, consistency is the key to developing and maintaining technical proficiency with the instrument. In Carroll's words, "Even if I'm not on tour, I play every day to keep my fingers in shape. If I'm short on time, only a few minutes are needed, but it's got to be every day. I learned the hard way when I once went on a holiday without a guitar. When I got home and tried to play, the strings felt like super high-tension cheese wire! It took another week to get back in shape and fully calibrated. Sometimes life throws things our way that make it hard to play every single day, but through these chapters, it's important to remember that even a little bit of playing and practice can go a long way."

Gordy agrees. "Playing a little every day is always better than a lot every few days or [once a] week. It's important to stay in tune with your instrument, just as your instrument needs to be in tune. And again, practice with a metronome—it will keep you honest."

Pascual offers, "Ideally, I try to practice for three different sessions every day. Even if those sessions are short, like 15 minutes, I've found that to be the best; if time permits, maybe one longer and two shorter sessions. If I'm playing concerts regularly, that pattern may change, but in periods of less frequent concerts or touring, I've found that three daily sessions is my goal. If that's not feasible, I try to keep the continuity by doing at least one or two sessions a day. After many years, I've discovered that daily consistency is way more important than the length of the sessions. Even a ten- or 15-minute session once or twice a day can go a long way to keeping your technique from declining."

For technical practice, de Grassi will start with something familiar and then focus on fundamentals. "I have a cross-string scale exercise I usually run through when I first sit down to play. Then I'll go over short difficult passages in my repertoire, scrutinize what I want to sound better, and then work on the micro details. Practice musical passages slowly, and focus on each aspect of technique—the timing, tone, dynamics, articulations, etc."

On Preparing for a Performance

All guitarists develop their own pre-show routine based on what works for them. But an overarching theme is to not overtax the hands or try to play music that is too difficult right before a performance, which can also have a detrimental effect on the psyche.

For Gordy, a big part of preparation is knowing that he is well-prepared—and subsequently letting go. "I don't practice anything in particular before a concert. If I'm feeling less confident about a tune or a passage that I'm playing that night, I'll try to keep it close to the surface of my mind and in my hands. But at some point, I have to just let it go and accept that I'm not going to get much better between now and the downbeat."

Vicki Genfan concurs. "If there are challenging passages in material I'll be performing, I like to run through those slowly and quietly before a gig. It's a balancing act. I want my muscle memory to be intact, but don't want to tire my fingers, arms, or hands." De Grassi adds, "I'll usually run through the difficult passages of the pieces I'm going to play, both at tempo and in slow motion. Get out front with your practicing at home so you're not cramming at the last minute."

Carroll suggests an honest approach, paired with the importance of being well-prepared and ultimately, enjoying the performance: "Sometimes I hit the record button on my phone and play a piece from the set list. The playback will soon give me an idea of how ready that piece really is! I'll usually write out a list of adjustments I'd like to make and get to work. The more prepared you are in advance of treading the boards, the more you'll enjoy delivering the music to your audience."

On Staying Healthy at Home or On the Road

Many professional guitarists tour regularly as part of their musical trajectories, and the demands of being on the road—international travel in particular—require thoughtful attention to sustaining good health and consistently high standards of performance.

Once again, Carroll emphasizes the merits of preparation. "These days, my tours usually follow an album release, and that recording is preceded by an intensive amount of attention to detail in the recording studio. Sometimes this preparation can feel like hell, but I sure am glad of all the prep work when I walk out onto the stage. Touring is quite exhausting most of the time, but it is also very enjoyable and addictive.

"After I've traveled for five hours or more and checked into the hotel, I know I should take in a 20-minute walk and eat a light salad but invariably, I'll lay down for 20 minutes and have a coffee and the hotel cookies instead! Before you know it, it's time to head to soundcheck. Eating late at night after the show used to be the norm, but these days, dinner is almost always before the show, and I feel much better the next day. The one thing I am a good boy about is stretching. In the mornings, it's all downward dog, angry cat legs, back, arms, fingers, neck: I do it all thanks to some tips from an expert a few years back. It really makes a difference for me—to the point where if I don't stretch, for whatever reason, I'll soon tighten up."

Genfan's preparation begins a month before her tours, starting with a daily practice routine based on her set lists, which may include new music or older tunes that need a refresh. She also prepares for the time on the road not on stage. "I always get all the supplies I'll need to stay healthy on the road well in advance," she says. "That usually includes vitamins, herbs, a yoga mat, or other exercise equipment, as well as downloading videos, music, podcasts, books, and plenty of healthy food and snacks."

When asked how else she stays healthy on the road—and at home—she offers, "It's simple—and sometimes very hard to do! Get enough sleep, eat good food, and get some regular exercise in. All these things can be greatly compromised when on the road, but eventually, if you don't tend to them, your body and mind will feel the consequences. If you have a meditation practice, that can be very helpful, as well. Whatever you can insert into your travel will be appreciated by your body and mind. Check out *holden-qigong.com* for a wonderful exercise practice you can do anywhere."

De Grassi recommends getting outside, especially when touring. "I always try to get out and walk as much as possible. That tends to release the nervous energy that accumulates from sitting on planes and in cars, and it helps set your diurnal clock when you're making time zone changes. Plus, I've always been interested in geography and urban design, and walking is the best way to discover something about where you are, even if it's some desolate Exit 19 along an interstate with a couple of hotels, a gas station, and a mini mall. I love observing civilization, and I'll often get ideas for new compositions while walking."

Juber makes sure he has the basics covered—extra strings, batteries, straps—and he consistently reviews his repertoire. He also emphasizes the benefits of a meditation practice, adding, "Stay hydrated, get some exercise, avoid carrying too much weight, sit at a desk when working on a laptop or pad, and limit alcohol!"

Gordy, who spent years on the road with the David Grisman Quintet, offers: "Touring is not easy. Depending on the schedule, it can feel like there's precious little free time just to move your body. So, take stretch breaks whenever you possibly can. Do a little yoga in the hotel room, and go for a run or a walk if there's time. Hydrate! Always, but especially when flying. Sometimes you just have to prioritize sleep, even when you miss the hang. Years ago, an older musician I was on tour with pointed out while we were backstage, surrounded by cheese plates and all the trappings of well-stocked green room hospitality, that we musicians are helping to create a special event that one night in that town/venue/theater—call it a party, if you like—but we can't live every day like it's a party. Balance is important, and so is personal sustainability."

On Creativity

The ability to stay creative and work through blocks is something that many musicians continually strive for. Songwriters are used to collaboration, and Genfan believes this practice can also help guitarists. "Collaboration is very powerful for me in terms of breaking out of ruts. I also love to challenge myself to recreate a song in another genre, like taking a folk song and arranging it in a reggae feel, or with an R&B feel. I have an exercise I often use to cultivate new ideas called 'rut busting.' I give myself two to five minutes when I first pick up my guitar, and I try to play things I've never played before; it's really about cultivating a mental state of 'anything goes.' I often do this in an open or alternate tuning, which is an exciting exercise—scales, patterns, or chords I may have played now sound completely new! I'll often record these exercises, and I always come across something cool, even if it's a small pattern, motif, or chord progression."

Carroll offers the following: "Writing or playing to a visual such as a painting or a video clip can really spark the imagination. Try picking out something random on YouTube such as horse riding in the wilderness, sailing to Antarctica, or the history of the music box—anything that takes your fancy, really. You only need about a minute's worth of video. Mute the sound and try to create music that fits the mood of the visual. You'll start to conjure sounds you never would have thought of by just staring at the fretboard and blank canvas alone."

Gordy adds, "Take a shower! Seriously, I've had some great breakthroughs in the shower when I'm stuck on a composing problem. Maybe it's the hot water on my brain. Sometimes seeking out other expressions can be helpful. Read a good book or spend an afternoon in a museum. Just getting out for a walk or a hike can give you some perspective. Don't discount exercise."

De Grassi will often spark his imagination by playing music from other genres or on another instrument. "Try playing something outside what you know, maybe even a different instrument. I keep a snare drum and hi-hat in my studio, and sometimes I sit at the piano and flip through the *Real Book*. Read through some sheet music you haven't looked at in years. Above all, keep listening to and learning new music. If you are bored, either go do something else or work on your technique."

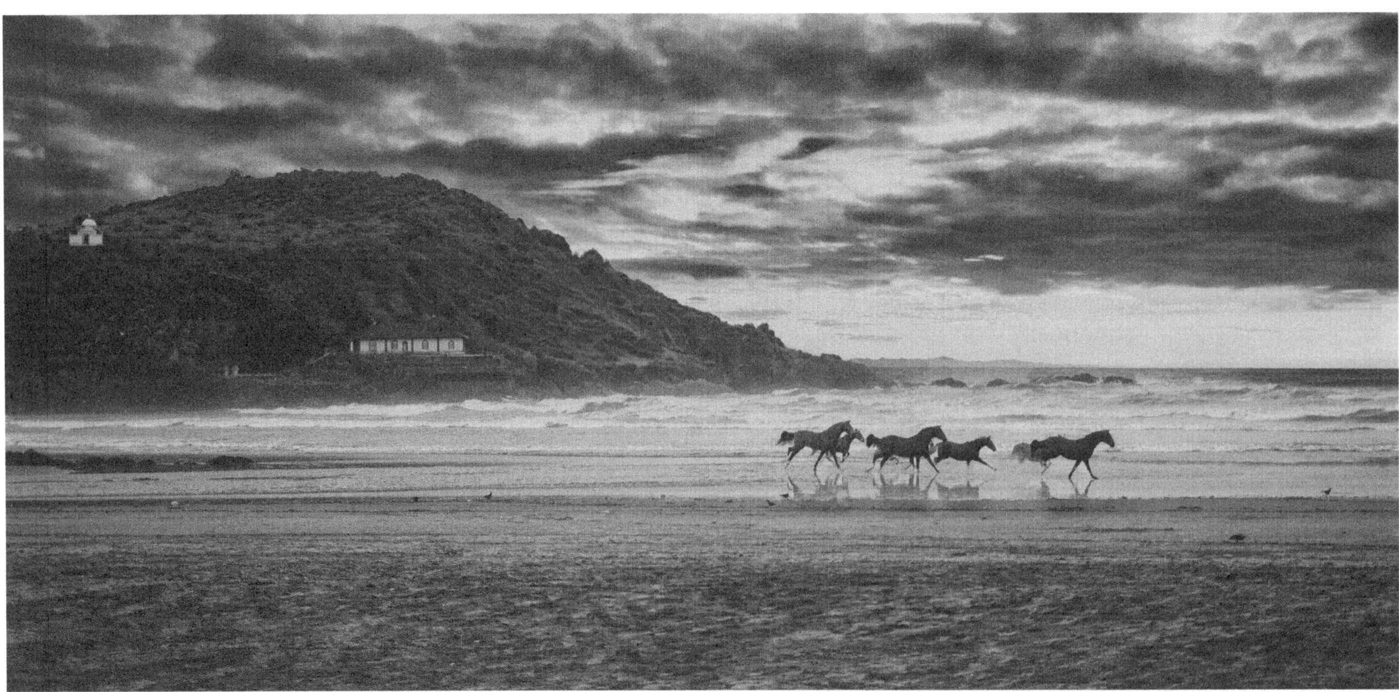

Using a guitar support, like Alex is here, allows both feet to be planted firmly on the ground.

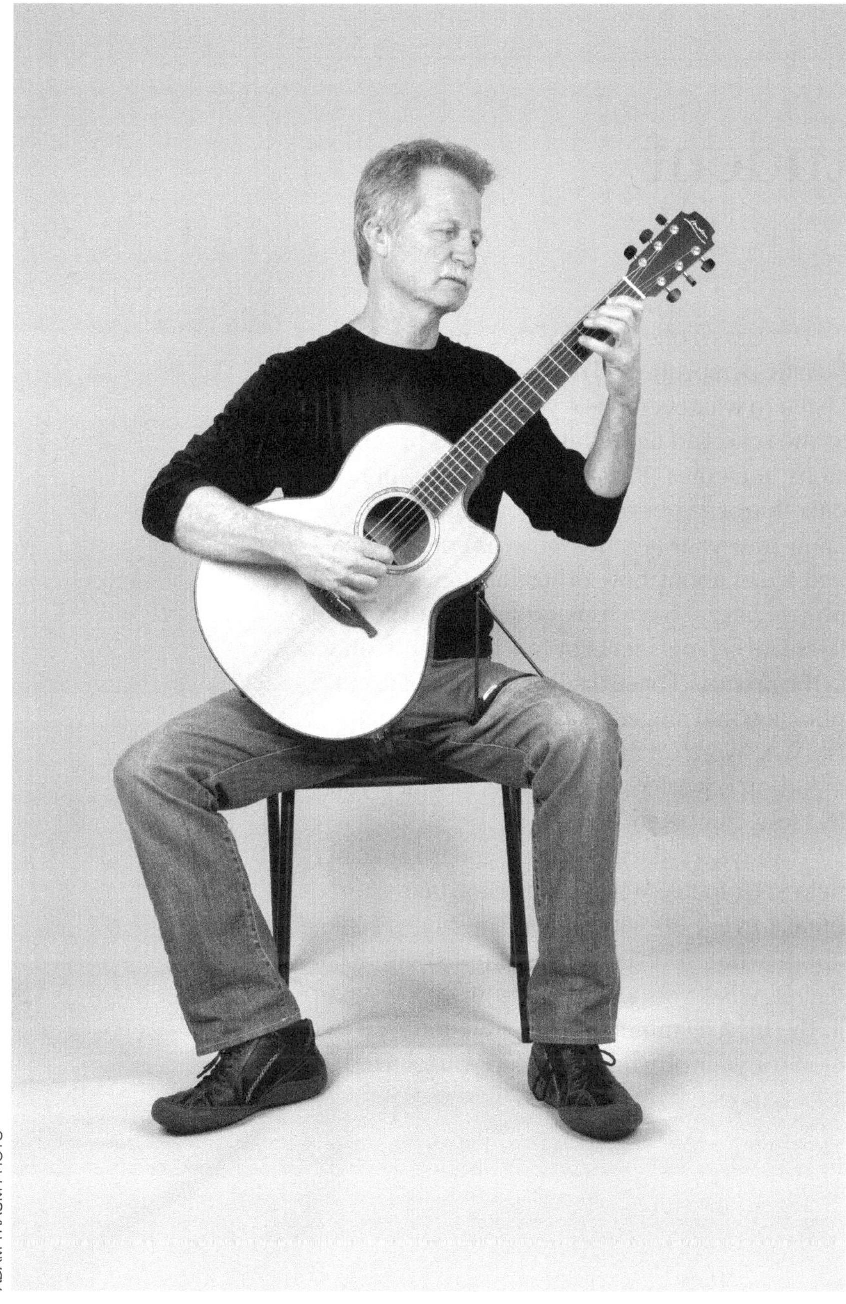

ADAM TRAUM PHOTO

On Guitar Posture

Most guitar players who have spent years performing and touring professionally have developed a sense of good guitar posture that promotes health and longevity, often integrating principles of ergonomics. Juber always uses a strap, even when sitting, which he credits for better posture.

Gordy suggests, "When I sit, I tend to hold the guitar between my knees, in a classical guitar style—not typical of a flatpicker, I know. It wasn't a conscious thing; I just like being able to angle the neck up a lot. When I stand, I hold it up fairly high. I came up playing a lot of bluegrass and bluegrass-adjacent music, and the big dreadnought guitar tends to be the standard axe for that setting, but I eventually switched to the 000 size because I realized it was more appropriate for my playing style, and I like the sound better."

Carroll adds, "I mostly sit when I play acoustic guitar. I use a footstool on its lowest setting, for the right foot. This eradicates any tension in that foot and beyond, and overall, the guitar sits comfortably. I used to play without the footstool, and I'd invariably end up using the chair leg as a support for my almost-vertical foot position."

"A basic guideline for me as someone who plays sitting down is to follow this simple procedure," offers Pascual. "Find a chair and sit in a position that is comfortable without the guitar. Keep both feet on the floor, spine straight, shoulders relaxed (not hunched), chin towards the chest to elongate the back of the neck, and breathe while you're relaxed. Then add the guitar without losing any comfort or compromising your relaxed breathing. Practice, but prioritize the comfort first, and see what happens. If you notice you are uncomfortable when you're holding the guitar, spend time getting your playing position with the guitar as comfortable as the non-playing position."

Genfan also pays close attention to her body throughout the practice session: "I'm a big proponent of mindfulness, and I always try to stay aware of how my body feels when I'm playing, particularly if and where I may be holding excessive tension. Whether I'm sitting or standing, I can always improve my experience by scanning my body and relaxing unwanted tension and/or moving the instrument or my body. Sometimes I use a footstool to avoid crossing my legs, and I'm looking into a guitar support device that many classical guitarists are using these days."

De Grassi adds, "Make sure the action on your guitar allows you to get the most volume and tone out of your guitar. If the action is too low, that will limit the potential for both volume and tone. Practice developing your sound on simple melodies and bass lines."

Advice to a New Student or Guitarist

When asked for advice to offer to a new student, Carroll believes in the importance of a good role model. "Find the right teacher for you. It's important to find someone who understands the crucial fundamentals of technique and can steer you along your musical path. Their inspiration and motivation, coupled with plenty of practice, will be the gateway to great fulfilment and enjoyment."

Gordy recommends a humble attitude and a regular diet of music appreciation. "Generally speaking, I think the most important thing is to humbly cultivate an ongoing fascination with music. Keeping love and interest foremost, noticing the effect good music has on your body and emotions, being open to new and unfamiliar styles, always trying to learn new things—tunes, rhythmic concepts, harmonic structures...We're so lucky to get to be music practitioners in the first place! And we can reflect that good fortune by attending to the music as deeply as possible. Pragmatically speaking, learning to read notation earlier on will save you a lot of time and anxiety in the future—especially if the goal is to play on a professional level."

Genfan underscores the importance of clarity. "Be clear about what you want. What are your musical goals? If you don't know, then you don't know what steps to take. Check in with yourself every six months or so to see what has changed or become clearer."

De Grassi offers advice that emphasizes a holistic perspective: "Transcribe music by ear. Listen to whatever music you are interested in at the time and figure out the chord progressions, melodies, bass lines, etc. You will not only sharpen your ears, but you will also get to know how your favorite music is constructed and learn about how other instrumentalists phrase lines. I have transcribed lots of songs to create arrangements or teach students, and in the process, I have discovered a lot of useful phrasing that singers and other instrumentalists use. Work on the skills that need improving—don't overlook those areas in which you feel less competent.

"Activities like meditation and tai chi can help your focus. When practicing, take short breaks every 20 minutes or half hour, think about what you've just accomplished, and decide what you are going to work on next in the next 30 minutes. That's a good way to monitor your practice and keep you focused."

In It for the Long Haul

All the guitarists featured throughout this book are exemplars of long-term—indeed, lifetime—dedication to music. Ultimately, what keeps all of us going is the love of playing guitar, plain and simple. Gratitude, patience, and perspective can really help in challenging moments, especially for professional musicians.

Gordy offers advice on staying positive and finding your own voice. "Stay positive amidst the challenges of being a musician. If you need inspiration, go see live music! It's all about love and patience. Be honest and critical but compassionate with yourself. It's hard to avoid being yourself if you're honest, which is a good thing. Always be open to new sounds, but also notice what moves you. Find a balance between emulating people whose playing you admire and moving closer to what you sound like. People have so many influences, and we all have a lot of deep influences that may not actually be audible in our playing. Above all else, music is fun. That's the goal—have fun!"

Genfan agrees. "*Listen* and imitate—that's how we did it in the old days! Find players whose sound you love. Experiment, record yourself, and listen back. Try to get some feedback from a teacher or player whose sound you love and admire. Write a lot and don't be afraid of writing bad compositions or songs! Listen to great music and go see live music whenever possible. Listen to music that you've recorded to remember the talents and gifts you have. There are also many inspiring podcasts and books. Listen and read—a lot!

"I've always adhered to the philosophy of following my joy. For me, that meant composing and playing in a niche category as an open-tuning guitarist. I haven't mastered many techniques that other guitarists use, such as improvising or chord melodies, but following my joy led me to create my own style and set of skills, of which I am very proud. They have allowed me to compose a lot of fun and unusual music—music that expresses my heart-songs. In general, I think music is a great gift, and if you lose the sense of fun and enjoyment as a player, it may be time to rethink your approach."

De Grassi also concurs. "Follow your instincts! Make whatever music you play a reflection of who you are. Try to remember—whether you are a professional, amateur, or student—that you started playing because you enjoy it. Playing guitar should always be fun."

Carroll summarizes: "Fundamentally, you need to enjoy playing. As an amateur golfer, I have no desire to become the next Rory McIlroy—my goal is to hit the ball straightish, that's all. At the same time, I listen to advice from people who are far better than I—almost everyone—with an open mind, and I listen to the pro who knows how to teach me that one thing that will enhance my game and make me feel inspired. I think the same applies for guitarists. Whether it's your profession or a hobby, make sure it stays enjoyable, and search out things that inspire you. Play with others, record yourself, and set realistic tasks. Maybe you might enjoy working up a few pieces to record for your family, or maybe it's an EP or full album for the store shelves. Whether it be strumming a song at your local folk club or performing the Rodrigo guitar concerto at Carnegie Hall, having direction and a goal is ultimately important."

On Preparing for a Tour

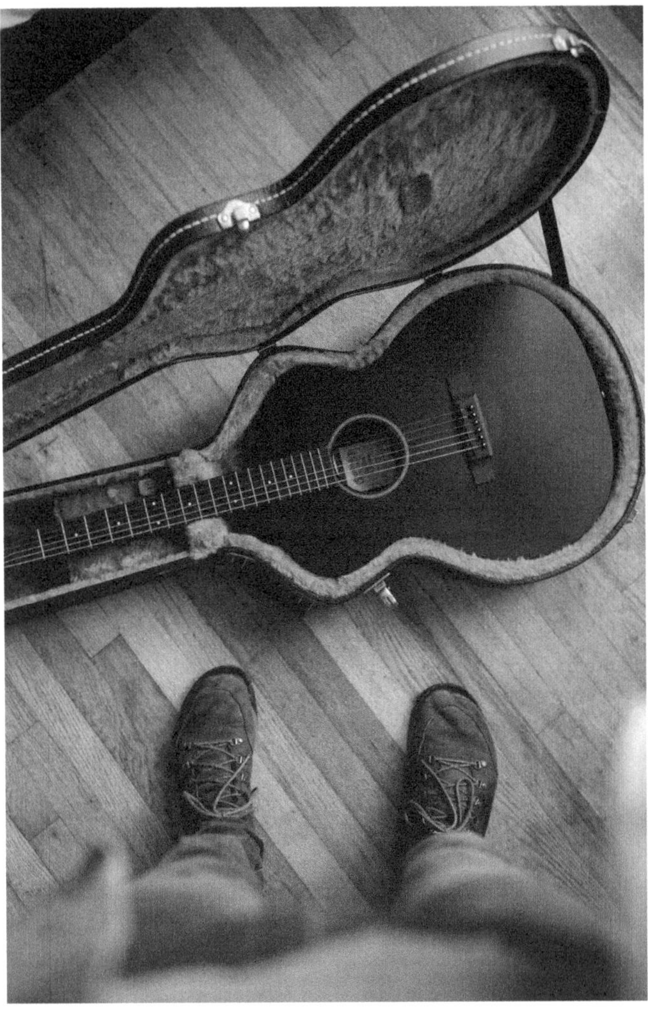

If you're new to touring, it's helpful to realize a tour consists of both musical and logistical facets. Being clear about these facets as separate endeavors helps to organize and manage everything. If you are an independent soloist, your role as performer expands to include roles critical to success: manager, agent, publicist, tour manager, musical director, and driver. In the case of the DIY band, these duties may fall on one person or be divided up amongst various band members. Being clear about and attending to all these as separate items is essential.

When preparing for the music and performance aspects, create and/or decide on repertoire, and schedule the necessary personal time to practice, as well as a full rehearsal if playing with a band. Be clear whether you're building a show or simply playing a set of songs. Creating a tight show requires extra preparation. There are many levels of this, of course, from deciding where in the program you're going to say a few words between pieces, to staging an entire production with lights, dancers, and choreography.

—Juanito Pascual

Logistics to Consider

Booking the concerts
Try to book venues and plan routes that work smoothly (avoiding unnecessary backtracking), prevent undesired days off, and minimize stress (like 12 hours in the car each day and a show every night).

Reviewing and signing contracts
Make sure that all details including payment and timing are clearly articulated in advance, in writing.

Promotion
This usually involves graphic design skills, videos, social media, writing a press release, and potentially working with your own publicist, in conjunction with the public relations teams at the venues.

Rehearsals
Coordinating rehearsals and travel schedules with the other musicians, especially if they change in different cities and venues.

Transportation and Lodging
Make sure to take care of this well in advance.

Technical needs
Contact each venue to confirm all sound reinforcement, equipment/backline, and other technical needs are in place, well in advance.

Budget
Establish a budget that accounts for everything, including gas, tolls, rental fees for vehicles and equipment, food and lodging for everyone on the tour, flights and luggage costs, as well as promotional costs. All these things need to be paid for, and not budgeting for them may leave you with little or no money to pay yourself and the other musicians.

Recording
Decide if you want to have your performances filmed and/or recorded. Secure a competent production team, or if you're doing everything yourself, make sure you have all the necessary equipment.

Recommended Reading

You Are Your Instrument: The Definitive Musician's Guide to Practice and Performance —Julie Lyonn Lieberman

The Art of Practicing: A Guide to Making Music from the Heart—Madeline Bruser

Effortless Mastery: Liberating the Master Musician Within—Kenny Werner

Touching Peace: Practicing the Art of Mindful Living —Thich Nhat Hahn

Being Peace—Thich Nhat Hahn

Kaizen: The Art of Transforming Habits, One Small Step at a Time—Sarah Harvey

Mastering the Art of Performance: A Primer for Musicians—Stewart Gordon

The Musician's Way: A Guide to Practice, Performance, and Wellness—Gerald Klickstein

Wabi Sabi: Japanese Wisdom for a Perfectly Imperfect Life—Beth Kempton

Wabi Sabi: The Wisdom in Imperfection—Nobuo Suzuki

The Alex de Grassi Fingerstyle Guitar Method—Alex de Grassi

Playing with Ease: A Healthy Approach to Guitar Technique—David Leisner

The Guitar Book—Pierre Bensusan

The Pierre Bensusan Guitar Collection—Pierre Bensusan

Rhythm, Sonority, Silence—Michael Hedges with John Stropes

About the Author

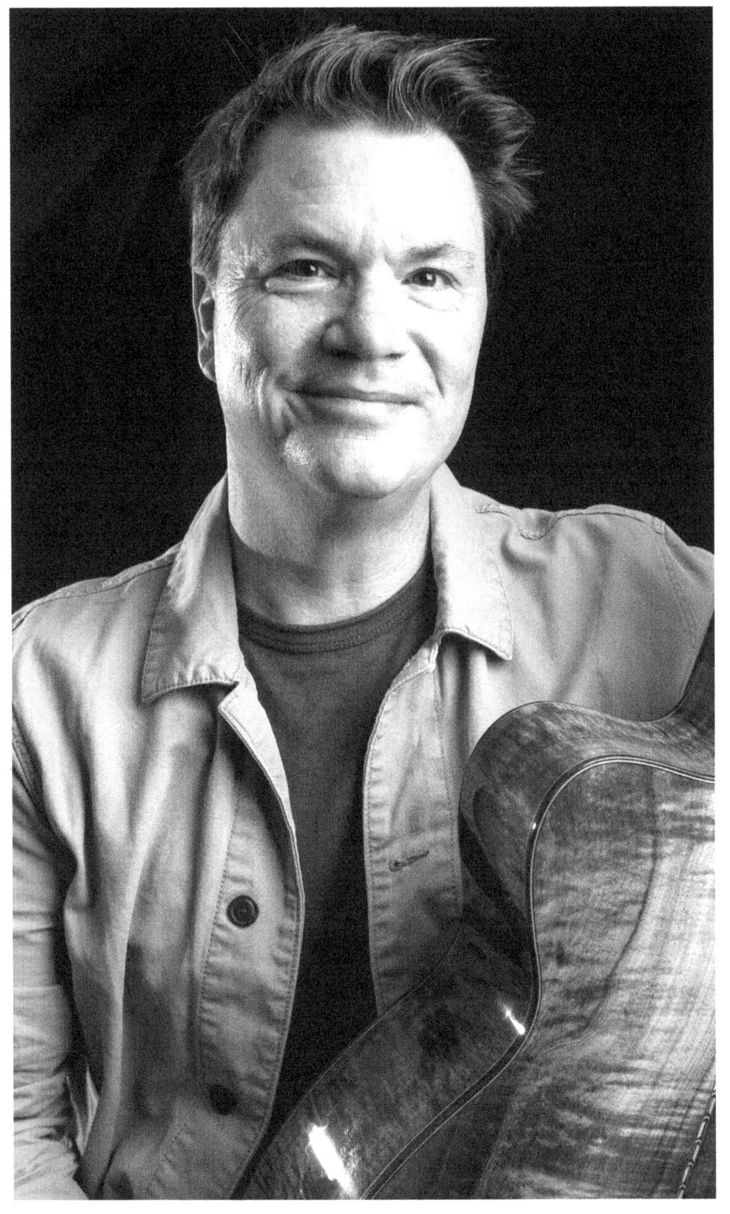

Sean McGowan is a strong advocate for injury prevention and health education for musicians, and his workshops incorporate a holistic approach to playing. As a fingerstyle jazz and acoustic guitarist, he combines many diverse musical influences with unconventional techniques to create a broad palette of textures within his compositions and arrangements for solo guitar. His recordings *Indigo* (2008) and *Sphere: the Music of Thelonious Monk* (2011) offer compelling portraits of jazz standards performed on solo electric archtop guitar. *Sphere* was named one of *Acoustic Guitar* magazine's "Essential Albums of 2011."

McGowan has been featured on the covers of *Fingerstyle 360, Jazz Guitar Today,* and *Fingerstyle Guitar Journal* magazines. His solo guitar recordings include *Thanksgiving & Christmas Tidings* (2014), a collection of seasonal hymns and carols arranged for acoustic guitar; *My Fair Lady* (2015), featuring tunes from the Broadway masterpiece; and *Union Station* (2022), with original compositions for jazz organ trio. His most recent recording is *Portmanteau* (2023), a set of timeless standards and songs from great American composers arranged for solo guitar.

As a performer and educator, McGowan has been featured at numerous jazz and guitar festivals, including the Swannanoa Guitar Week, Alex de Grassi's Mendocino Guitar Workshop, Nashville Fingerstyle Guitar Retreat, Frank Vignola's Big Jersey Guitar, Artisan, La Conner, Rocky Mountain Archtop, Healdsburg, Novi Sad Jazz, and many others. In 2021, McGowan performed and taught for the GFA International Convention, one of the few jazz guitarists to ever be invited to perform and teach.

McGowan currently serves as a professor of music for the Music & Entertainment Industry Studies department at the University of Colorado Denver, one of the largest contemporary music programs in the United States. He earned a DMA in guitar performance from the University of Southern California in Los Angeles and has conducted workshops at colleges and guitar organizations throughout the country.

McGowan contributes lesson content to *Acoustic Guitar* magazine and is the author of *Fingerstyle Jazz Guitar Solos* (Hal Leonard) and the String Letter Media book/video instruction methods *The Acoustic Jazz Guitarist, Fingerstyle Jazz Guitar Essentials,* and *Holiday Songs for Fingerstyle Guitar*. He has also produced over a dozen courses for TrueFire, covering the topics of fingerstyle jazz, improvisation, and comping.
seanmcgowanguitar.com

About the Guest Contributors

Clive Carroll is a luminary among contemporary steel-string fingerstyle guitarists. Born in England, Carroll earned a degree in composition and classical guitar from Trinity College in London, and subsequently met John Renbourn, who took Carroll on the road with him for tours throughout Europe and North America. A prolific recording and performing artist, Carroll has worked with John Williams, Tommy Emmanuel, Xuefei Yang, Ralph Towner, D'Gary, and Vishwa Mohan Bhatt, among many others. **clivecarroll.co.uk**

Since his debut on Windham Hill records in the 1970s, **Alex de Grassi** has long been considered one of the leading musical architects of modern steel-string fingerstyle guitar. He has toured internationally for the past 40 years and has composed and recorded many seminal works for solo guitar and ensemble, earning a Grammy nomination for his album *The Water Garden*. He is the author of *The Alex de Grassi Fingerstyle Guitar Method* (String Letter Media). **degrassi.com**

A longtime fixture in the Pacific Northwest jazz scene, **Mike Doolin** is also noted as an innovative and forward-thinking luthier for nylon-string, steel-string, archtop, and harp guitars. As a luthier, he has presented at the Roberto-Venn School of Lutherie, the American School of Lutherie, and the Guild of American Luthiers Conventions. He has built instruments for Muriel Anderson, John Stowell, and Esperanza Spaulding, and recorded several albums with various artists as a seven-string guitarist. **doolinguitars.com**

Vicki Genfan is an award-winning fingerstyle guitarist noted for her innovative techniques and tunings, utilized in service of her recordings of original music and mesmerizing concert performances. As a singer-songwriter, she draws inspiration from pop, jazz, world, folk, and soul music, and is a frequent guest educator at music festivals such as the Swannanoa Gathering Guitar Week. Genfan has several instructional courses on developing rhythm, tunings, and fingerstyle techniques available through TrueFire. **vickigenfan.com**

A longtime guitarist for the David Grisman Quintet, **Grant Gordy** is widely considered an innovative and leading voice of flatpicking guitar and newgrass music. His solo recordings run from straight-ahead jazz and progressive acoustic string band music with top musicians such as Alex Hargreaves and Dominick Leslie to an acclaimed duo recording, *Year of the Dog*, with guitarist Ross Martin. Grant has recorded and performed with the acoustic supergroup Mr. Sun and was featured on the cover of *Acoustic Guitar* magazine in 2023. **grantgordy.com**

A prolific and award-winning fingerstyle guitarist, **Mark Hanson** has recorded numerous solo acoustic guitar albums (including the Grammy-winning *Pink Guitar* compilation of Henry Mancini compositions) and has authored over two dozen highly acclaimed instructional books and DVD courses. A graduate of Stanford University, Hanson served as the senior editor for *Frets* magazine in the 1980s, interviewing top acoustic artists such as James Taylor, David Crosby, and Leo Kottke. **markhansonguitar.com**

With an international career recording and touring for over four decades, **Eric Johnson** is considered one of the most influential guitarists of our time, seamlessly blending influences of rock, country, jazz, pop, classical, and blues to create an instantly recognizable and personal sound. His seminal, platinum-certified album *Ah Via Musicom* won a Grammy award for the guitar standard "Cliffs of Dover." Johnson has been featured on the cover of several guitar publications, including *Acoustic Guitar* magazine, and has toured exclusively as a solo acoustic performer. **ericjohnson.com**

Internationally recognized as the guitarist for Wings with Paul McCartney, **Laurence Juber** has recorded over two dozen acoustic guitar albums showcasing his deft fingerstyle technique and mastery of composition and arranging pop standards. His album *LJ Plays the Beatles* is considered an essential solo guitar recording, and his contributions to the album *Pink Guitar* earned him a Grammy award. He has authored several books, including *The Evolution of Fingerstyle Guitar* (Hal Leonard) and has composed original scores for numerous television, film, theatre, and video game projects, including the award-winning game *Diablo III*. **laurencejuber.com**

Kyle Knuppel, M.D., is a board-certified medical doctor with degrees in voice performance and composition from Berklee College of Music. As a physician, he has years of experience lending clinical expertise to emergency room treatment throughout rural America, overseeing hospitals and care centers in India and Africa, and leading neurorehabilitation endeavors internationally. He is currently the Director of Clinical Innovation, providing administrative and clinical expertise to address health disparities among Indigenous and Alaskan Native communities throughout the United States.

Jeff LaQuatra is an award-winning classical guitarist and director of the guitar performance program at Colorado State University in Fort Collins, Colorado. A former student of Ricardo Iznaola, his debut recording, *Twilight: Guitar Music at the End of the Century*, was released by Iznaola Guitar Works. As a chamber musician, he has performed with the Boulder Philharmonic Orchestra and Central City Opera. He is currently a member of Quatra Duo, recording newly commissioned works and touring the United States and China. **libarts.colostate.edu/people/jefflaq**

Equally at home traversing jazz, pop, and acoustic styles, **Adam Levy** is a highly regarded session and touring guitarist, songwriter, and educator. Levy has recorded and performed with Lizz Wright, Norah Jones, and Tracy Chapman, among many others. The host of the popular *Guitar Tips with Adam Levy*, he is also the author of *String Theories: Tips, Challenges, and Reflections for the Lifelong Guitarist* with Ethan Sherman. **adamlevy.com**

Juanito Pascual is an acclaimed flamenco guitarist based in Minneapolis. He is the author of *The Total Flamenco Guitarist* (Alfred) and performs and teaches workshops regularly throughout the United States, Europe, and Central America. Pascual was trained at the New England Conservatory of Music in Boston, and his original compositions and recordings reflect the intersections of flamenco traditions with jazz, improv, and world music. He is an ongoing collaborator with Earth Train, a Panamanian rainforest project that uses music and art as a means to inspire and educate a new generation about environmental stewardship. **juanitopascual.com**